The
Morning
Sickness
Companion

The
Morning
Sickness
Companion

by Elizabeth Kaledin

ST. MARTIN'S GRIFFIN ❧ THOMAS DUNNE BOOKS
NEW YORK

THOMAS DUNNE BOOKS.
An imprint of St. Martin's Press.

www.stmartins.com

Design by The Book Design Group

Photographs printed with permission by Cathy Claman, copyright © 2002.
The model in the photographs is Kristin Campbell.

ISBN 0-312-28489-6

First Edition: April 2003

10 9 8 7 6 5 4 3 2 1

For Noelle and Tobias, who were worth every
minute of the misery

And for Jon, the best "morning sickness
companion" I could have hoped for

Contents

Contents

Acknowledgments

Writing this book, I often joke, was just like the experience of having a third child. There was conception, nine months and more of growth and development, and an extremely difficult labor and delivery. And, of course, I experienced plenty of nausea along the way, wondering why in the world I had taken on this project on the heels of having a new baby and going back to work, and if I could get it done.

In the end I did manage to "give birth" to a book I hope will benefit women, but it only happened with the assistance and encouragement of many "mid-wives" along the way. First, my great friend, author Mary Jane Clark: I vividly remember sitting across from her at lunch one day, feeling wretched as usual, and complaining about the dearth of books on the subject of morning sickness. I outlined *my* idea for a book and her enthusiasm instantly transformed a vague notion in my head into a realistic goal. She hooked me up with her own agent and sent me on my way. It's safe to say that without Mary Jane and her advice, support, and friendship, this book never would have been written.

My husband and steadfast companion, Jon Dohlin, is another reason this book was written. He never made it anything other than a foregone conclusion that it could be done, and he was a constant source of ideas, inspiration, and love.

In the advice at the end of the book, my sister-in-law Christine Horigan writes that everyone suffering morning sickness should find a "kindred spirit to comfort them." She was that person for me. As a fellow morning sickness sufferer, she knew exactly what I was going through, and her commiseration, friendship, and ability to laugh and cry at the situation in the same breath pulled me through and gave me courage on more days than I can count.

My other sister-in-law, Cathy Claman, was another never-ending source of sympathy and support, and she volunteered her time and expert eye to take the photographs in the chapter on exercise.

My brothers, Nicholas and Jonathan, cheered me on with their support and pride, and never gave me a hard time, as brothers can do sometimes, about the strange things I was eating.

Coming from the world of broadcast journalism, which

requires a distinct style of writing, I needed a lot of help navigating the publishing world, and my agent, Laura Dail, was patient and generous with her time and advice. She gave me the confidence to write in my own voice instead of a preconceived notion of how a book should sound.

CBS researcher Debbie Rubin was instrumental in helping me gather what little information there was about morning sickness, and she checked all my facts as diligently as she checks the facts delivered on the *CBS Evening News with Dan Rather*.

Pregnancy exercise expert Peggy Levine donated her time and expertise to a careful reading of the chapter on exercise, making sure all the suggested stretches are safe. She also found our model Kristin, who was willing to be photographed in the poses the day before she delivered her son.

Of course, I owe a debt of gratitude to all the women who patiently filled out my survey. Many of them struggled to do it while they were feeling awful, and their voices and their honesty I believe bring the most value to this book.

And finally, I want to thank my parents. My father, Arthur Kaledin, was one of my earliest enthusiasts and editors. He supported the idea from the start, and carefully read my manuscript, filling its margins with dozens of comments and suggestions that became incorporated into the final product. And my mother, Eugenia Kaledin, has always taught me to appreciate the beauty of the English language and the value of a clear, well-written sentence. Thank you both for so much guidance, wisdom, and love.

Foreword

Morning sickness. We still have no idea what to do about it. As a doctor, I am fascinated by how little we have progressed in terms of treating this pervasive pregnancy problem. We can do so many amazing things for pregnant women and their unborn fetuses and yet we can't get rid of that miserable nausea, vomiting, and overwhelming fatigue. On the one hand, it isn't dangerous; it has no ill effect on the fetus or the mother, it almost always dissipates after the first trimester, and it probably has biological significance, maybe even survival advantage. Unfortunately, that doesn't really help you when you're so miserable that you can't crawl out of bed or let go of the toilet seat.

Having been there and done that, I am quite sympathetic toward my patients who suffer with it, and we always spend a good deal of time at our first meeting discussing it—why it occurs, what to try to do about it, and when it should be over. I find that while I rarely offer great solutions to my patients' symptoms, many women really just want to know that what they are experiencing is normal, that they aren't harming their babies, and that it will go away. Empathy goes a very long way, and people are always thrilled to hear that I went through it as well. I think people feel that doctors are immune to the everyday occurrences of pregnancy and cannot relate to their feelings, but we sure can.

It's important to emphasize that morning sickness is normal. It is normal to lose your excitement about the pregnancy. It is normal to worry about and yet resent being pregnant, and it is normal to wish you weren't. The moment your appetite returns and you can keep your eyes open, you truly forget you were ever sick. The symptoms can vary enormously from woman to woman, but it is very often present in some form. It may be as innocuous as a small amount of queasiness once a day, to pervasive nausea and vomiting requiring hospitalization, intravenous hydration, and rarely, intravenous feedings. It usually goes away. It is the rare patient who is still very symptomatic after twelve to fourteen weeks. Women with twins may experience longer bouts due to their more exaggerated elevations in pregnancy hormone beta HCG (Human Chorionic Gonadotropin).

The important thing to keep in mind is that it is almost unheard of for a fetus to suffer adverse effects from morning sickness, *regardless* of the degree. This is one of the things potential moms worry about consistently. Am I hurting the baby? They are not. Husbands sometimes worsen the mothers' anxiety by pestering them to eat more even when they cannot, and reinforcing their fears about harm to their fetus. Educating the fathers-to-be helps a lot, and allays fears. The fetus in the first trimester is tiny. It is less than a few centimeters long and can thrive on maternal nutrient stores even if Mom is eating poorly, or often not at all. For those women considering pregnancy in the near future, we always advise them to start prenatal vitamins early so that in the event they do experience debilitating symptoms, they have plenty of nutrients in storage to feed their fetus. A mother may become somewhat depleted of nutrients after a pregnancy, but the baby usually thrives at her expense! Moreover, most women will feel better after twelve weeks of gestation, and they can easily make up for lost weight and nutrition later in pregnancy. It is amazing how quickly one forgets the misery of the first trimester once one is eating again. On the contrary, women who are malnourished prior to pregnancy and suffer severe nausea could have poor intrauterine growth later in gestation and should be watched carefully.

We try to encourage women who suffer from severe nausea to eat anything that stays down. It is important to remember that calories in any form are far more important than balancing your diet in early pregnancy. If you eat what is right for you and it comes back up, it gives you no benefit. Eat the things that stay down, even if they are not what you envisioned. Also; stay hydrated. Dehydration may put you in the hospital; even though that isn't a terrible thing, and it's often short-term, it can be very upsetting, especially to a woman with other children at home. Again, drink what stays down, even if it's nothing but cola or ginger ale.

There are several antiemetic (antinausea) medications available for use in pregnancy. If you find that you are debilitated to a point that you cannot tolerate, speak with your doctor about them. We use them quite often and are comfortable with their safety. There are very few things that can harm you or your baby. Don't experiment with medication however, unless your physician approves it. Again, there are antinausea medications that are safe in pregnancy, but your doctor should discuss them with you. If you have any uncertainty regarding any foods, natural remedies, or medications, again, always check them out first. Some of the medications can be administered rectally for those patients who are truly bringing up everything.

Try the things your friends recommend. Although we obviously do not have any cure-alls for morning sickness, some of the common recommendations are based on loose facts and experience. The most likely things that offer help are the carbohydrate-containing foods like potatoes, bagels, breads, plain pastas, and crackers. There is something to this; it's not a panacea. There is some emerging evidence that ginger works. Whether it's in the form that one gets with sushi, or in ginger ale, or in ginger snaps (my personal favorite), it seems to provide some relief. Syrup from cola is soothing to the stomach as well. The small amount of caffeine won't hurt you. If you're that nause-ated, the amount you'll consume won't do anything harmful. Studies confirm that up to three caffeine-containing products per day in any trimester is safe. There is also some evidence that B-6 or B-complex vitamins may help. As the B vitamins are water-soluble and not stored by the body, you will often excrete the extra that you don't use.

It can be hard to work at a job during the first trimester, especially if you suffer from nausea and exhaustion. Even the most understanding employer still needs you functioning. Try to sleep whenever you can; you may not feel rested, but it is doing you some good. Also, pray that your boss is pregnant when you are. Try to keep in mind a few critical things. All these miserable symptoms are probably biologically important and may even offer survival advantages from centuries ago when man was primitive. People with the most trying symptoms have often been shown to have the healthiest pregnancies. This probably reflects higher levels of the pregnancy hormone HCG. Unhealthy pregnancies in the uterus and ectopic pregnancies often have lower levels of HCG and produce fewer bad symptoms. As a physician, I always feel a bit of anxiety when one of our patients tells us how great she is feeling, until I can confirm on ultrasound that the pregnancy is viable.

While it is *absolutely normal* to feel well in the first trimester, sometimes it can be a sign of an unhealthy pregnancy.

On the other hand, when I see someone holding an emesis bag, with that all-too-familiar pallor and expression of exasperation, I smile, for I know they're going to have a good pregnancy. I remember being in their shoes like it was yesterday. Keep in mind that you will get better. It is a rare patient who suffers past the late first trimester. If you do, however, speak to your doctor, as there are other conditions that may cause your nausea to persist and may need to be addressed. Most important, you will not hurt your baby! Do what you need to do to get through this and don't let other people discourage you. Try different things and experiment. I promise you, if you ask around, you will be hard-pressed to find anyone whose baby suffered as a result of morning sickness. My two beautiful, intelligent sons, Josh and Jake, are testimony to the fact that all a fetus needs in the first trimester is seven hundred mashed potatoes and a good toilet seat for Mom to cling to.

Ah, that brings me to my pregnancy. I was one of the lucky ones; the morning sickness was over and done with by twelve weeks. But let me tell you what a long twelve weeks that was. I thought it would never end. All the excitement I felt at seeing my positive pregnancy test went straight out the window and all I could do was think about how absolutely miserable I was for all my waking hours. I remember finding out I was pregnant the day my period was due. (How neurotic can you be, right?) I was so excited, and I remember telling my husband Ricky, who is also an obstetrician-gynecologist, how great I felt and how I was going to be one of those lucky women who sailed through pregnancy without a hint of nausea. Then six and a half weeks came along. You do wonder where the misnomer "morning sickness" comes from. I was queasy all day and all night. My only relief was during sleep, which I found I could do for over thirteen hours each night and wake still feeling thoroughly exhausted. The sad thing was that I rarely vomited. I just felt like I needed to all day long. I thought if only I could, maybe I'd feel better. I once stuck my fingers down my throat in desperation, only to gag and find that there really wasn't anything in there to come up anyway.

I listened in rapt attention to anyone who would tell me something that had worked for her, and then I'd make one of the poor nurses in my office run out to buy whatever it was, only to find that it barely helped, if at all. My best relief came in the form of mashed potatoes. I ate them by the truckload. I'd come home at night and Ricky would be mashing away and ask me how many I thought I could get down. Six to eight was typical. Did I eat protein? Fish? Eggs? Meat? Oh, no; nor vegetables, nor fruits. Everything tasted strange or awful to me, so I gave up trying to eat what I thought I should eat and ate what stayed down. I, with the stomach of steel, the one who can eat week-old spoiled food and be clueless, was thinking everything had gone bad. So I ate mashed potatoes. I think I ate a banana once, but I'm not sure. The thought of my prenatal vitamins made me retch. Even the smell sent a wave of nausea through me, and I put them far back in the cabinet until after sixteen weeks. I had the distinct advantage of being an obstetrician, with more knowledge about morning sickness than the average person, so I really knew I didn't have to worry about the baby; I just tortured everyone around me with how utterly miserable I was.

My sister-in-law recommended Atomic Fire Balls— those red, jawbreaker-like sucking candies. She swore they instantly took her nausea away. I tried, no success; although my eyes watered like crazy. One patient of mine said that Granny Smith apples did it for her. I never made it through a single one. I tried anything and everything. I hounded my poor patients for advice and suggestions. Needless to say, they were quite disheartened to learn that I, who was supposed to hold all the magical answers, was as hopeless as they were. I kept bagels and bagel chips in each exam room in my office and nibbled all day long. As bad as the nausea was, and as lousy as my appetite was, I found it was ten times worse if my stomach was empty, so I ate nonstop. I had the great fortune of putting on seventeen pounds in my first trimester, all from potatoes and bagels. How unfair was that?

Adding insult to injury, I was profoundly exhausted. I'd crawl home at five o'clock and say to Ricky, "I'm just going to rest for a few minutes." He'd wake me for my potatoes and then I'd crash until 6:00 A.M., when I had to get up again. When the alarm clock went off, I couldn't get out of bed. I was dead! I couldn't believe the night was over. I'd drag myself to work without a smudge of makeup (you'd have to know me to realize the implications of *that*), hating everyone and everything. Then I'd sit in my office and pray for patients to cancel their appointments so I could nap on my desk. The poor, unfortunate patients who did keep their appointments would be subjected to a barrage of my miseries. I think I spent more time complaining to patients than listening to them during my pregnancy. It was truly pathetic.

Elizabeth Kaledin has written a wonderful book that is an indispensable guide for any pregnant woman suffering with morning sickness. While it may not make you better, at least you'll know you are not alone, and while you may be feeling awful, it is all worth it for that incredible gift arriving only a few months from now. Best of luck to you. That first trimester will end, I promise.

—Lynn S. Friedman, M.D.
New York, NY

Introduction: Why Am I Writing This Book?

Early on in my second pregnancy, I announced to my obstetrician that I had started to throw up every day and was feeling downright subhuman. I felt unable to work, incapable of caring for my little girl, and though all thoughts of food made me ill, all I wanted to do was to eat. The dreaded "morning sickness" had taken hold. On hearing my bad news, my doctor smiled and chirped *"Mazel Tov!"* Now, I love my obstetrician, but I confess I *did* want to kill him at that moment. As I sat there glumly steeling myself for three to four months of the worst kind of nausea and vomiting and abject misery, he was merrily congratulating me.

That juxtaposition of feelings captured the paradox of morning sickness for me: few people ever really dwell on the trauma of it, because it is the famous first sign of a glorious occasion to come—the birth of a child.

In fact, most if not all doctors consider morning sickness the sign of a healthy pregnancy, a tangible indication that an embryo has firmly implanted itself in the uterine lining and is set to go! So the accompanying sickness is brushed aside. "It'll pass," they all say. "It's just a temporary and necessary evil of pregnancy," others chime in. "You'll forget all about it when the baby comes."

All of those things are true. But there is another truth about morning sickness that is rarely discussed with as much enthusiasm. For those of us who suffer through it, it can be positively debilitating, depressing, and alienating. Baby or no baby.

For four solid months during my second pregnancy, I was as sick and miserable as I have ever been in my life. At home, I practically wore out a spot on the rug in front of the toilet as I knelt there, sometimes throwing up over and over again, sometimes wishing I could throw up over and over again. At one point, my three-year-old daughter Noelle got so concerned about seeing me there that she came into the bathroom, rubbed my back, and in an attempt to comfort me, said, "Don't worry, Mommy. Everyone has problems!"

Boy, did I have problems. Anything could make me sick at any time of day or night. My husband Jon helplessly asked day after day if there was anything he could do to make it go away, and the exasperating, devastating answer was "NO."

I would drag myself in to work relieved that I had even been able to shower and dress, only to shut myself in my office, where I would throw up in my wastebasket and collapse on my couch. Thank God I had a couch.

When I felt I could eat, I ate like an animal, stealthily wolfing down meals I scarcely tasted. For weeks, I ate all alone, avoiding meals with friends because eating had become such a bizarre combination of obsession, chore, and treatment. I ate the same bland, comfort foods over and over again, hoping they would bring relief. For one week, it was white rice and peas. Another week, it was canned pears. If I didn't get my turkey-and-cheese sandwich from the Blimpie around the corner at the very *dot* of noon, I would start to shake. I ate an entire container of pineapple in the grocery store even before paying for it, and inhaled graham crackers as though they were oxygen itself. Yet the woman who loves salads, tofu, and healthy fresh produce couldn't even look at a vegetable. I was a mess.

Then there was work.

As a television journalist, my job involves going out in the field to interview people, getting on planes, and meeting deadlines. All of these tasks that I had been doing for years became the equivalent of climbing Mount Everest barefoot. I threw up in the middle of interviews, suddenly ripping off my microphone and running out of the room. I had to tell camera crews they had five minutes to light and shoot my "on-camera" stand-up because I knew I was going to get sick. Sure enough, as soon as I was done, I would bolt to the nearest bathroom with not a moment to spare. I wanted to do it after being on-camera because throwing up made my eyes water, my makeup run, and my nose turn red. So glamorous! I dreaded being far away from my office, my wastebasket, and my couch, and of course I was filled with the added anxiety of not performing my job to the best of my ability. Stomachache on top of stomachache!

My purse, once full of newspapers and notebooks, was now stuffed with crackers, warm cans of Coke, and hard candy because I was afraid to be without them. I felt like a freak and came to dread the simplest tasks because I felt so weary and vulnerable. Let's face it: no matter how understanding other people may be, throwing up in public is humiliating.

Friends were sympathetic; some had been through it themselves. But I discovered that despite all the sympathy, feeling nauseous twenty-four hours a day for weeks on end is an utterly lonely, dehumanizing, and desperate experience. Having to look good and put-together on-camera for a living made it all the worse.

For comfort, I turned to books, and to my profound disappointment, I found that the dizzying array of pregnancy guides at the bookstore gave the subject short shrift. I would find at most two pages, usually one paragraph, and always the same maddening refrain:

EAT CRACKERS

EAT SMALL MEALS

EAT CARBOHYDRATES BEFORE GOING TO SLEEP

AVOID GREASY FOODS

TRY POWDERED GINGER

In her 430-page book *The Complete Guide to Pregnancy*, Sheila Kitzinger offers two meager paragraphs on morning sickness, saying:

> If you suffer from morning sickness, a cup of tea and a few crackers or dry toast on waking may prevent it, or crackers alone may be better.

Not to single out Sheila, but I had to wonder, was she kidding? Had any of these people pushing crackers and toast—and ginger, of all things—ever actually spoken to a woman suffering with morning sickness? A woman who can barely ingest toast, let alone something as potent and strong-tasting as ginger?

And my favorite bit of useless advice the books offer over and over again is this: "Be sure to take good care of your teeth, visit the dentist, brush and floss regularly, because if you're throwing up, all that stomach acid could harm your teeth." Now, I'm all for white, shiny teeth, but during my bout with morning sickness, I could barely put a toothbrush in my mouth, and the *last* thing on my mind was, "Gee, I better get to the dentist!"

I felt like *screaming* when I read these books. Why wasn't anybody addressing the emotional and physical toll morning sickness takes? Why wasn't anybody writing about how hard it is to work or to care for a small child when you're on the verge of throwing up all day long? Why doesn't anyone share first-person accounts of what they've eaten or the crazy things they've tried just to make themselves feel better? Wasn't there anything more to say than . . . *crackers*?

Since crackers obviously weren't doing the trick for me, I was hungry for some other support system and found none . . . and the idea for this book was born. Actually, the idea was born at my prenatal exercise class, where I met a woman who confided in me that she couldn't brush her teeth because of her morning sickness. Eureka! I had the same problem! Every time I put a toothbrush in my mouth, I had an instant gag reflex. I tried to brush anyway because, well, it's a slippery slope toward becoming a complete social outcast when you give up toothbrushing. But it was a daily struggle, and I felt depressed and embarrassed about it. But when I met someone who had the same struggle and we could talk, and *laugh* about it, I instantly felt better.

Since there is no great body of scientific literature or knowledge out there about morning sickness, other women and their experiences, I discovered, are the finest remedy available for the desperation and loneliness accompanying this travail. Talking to other women made me realize that, yes, it *is* hard to get through the day, *no one* eats the perfect diet, *no one* gains the requisite twenty-five pounds, and it's *all* about survival. The sooner you eat what you want, I learned, the sooner you'll feel better. My sister-in-law Christine popped a Lean Cuisine frozen entrée into the microwave at ten o'clock every morning because a full, hot meal was the only thing that could carry her from breakfast to lunch. My best friend Mary Jane ate a Whopper with cheese every single day for six months because it made her feel better. Another lived on mashed potatoes. Another on fresh-squeezed orange juice. And I, contrary to conventional wisdom, couldn't stand the thought of ginger ale and opted instead for gallons and gallons of icy-cold skim milk. In the neurotic delirium that pregnancy can evoke, I felt compelled to interrogate my doctor about the potential for calcium poisoning. He smiled politely and said not to worry.

Speaking of doctors, you will read three words often in this book: ASK YOUR DOCTOR. That's because there is little proof, little evidence, and no years and years of scientific research behind any of the remedies for morning sickness. There's been no randomized, double-blind, placebo-controlled study of the effect of crackers on nausea. So much of what we know or believe works is anecdotal, and when it comes to protecting your safety and the safety of your baby, it's best just to be sure that your doctor knows and approves of what you're doing.

My point in this book is to impart what little knowledge there is on the subject and to combine it with the experiences and experiments of other women. I believe we can learn from each other. To that end, I drafted a morning-sickness questionnaire that I distributed to hundreds of women: friends, strangers, friends of friends, sisters of friends, mothers of friends, anyone who would listen. Sprinkled throughout these pages then, you will find those survey answers about everything from strange food cravings to feelings about life at the time. They are first-person accounts from the front lines of morning sickness, and it's these voices filled with humor, despair, and honesty that you will find most useful. As I read over all the question-

naires I received, I often wished I could invite all these
women over for tea because they were so comforting, and
my hope is that they, in their indirect way, can become *your*
morning-sickness companions. I want you to know that
even when you feel your worst, you are not alone: Someone
else is subsisting on cheeseburgers, drinking warm Coke at
9:00 A.M., and barfing on the bus. And crying about it
despite the undeniable joy of knowing a baby is on the way.

Short of a cure for morning sickness, a cure *not* on the
horizon, we might as well search for better ways to survive
it. I believe that means turning to each other to share our
trials, tribulations, and of course, all of our remarkable
strengths.

The
Morning
Sickness
Companion

1

So You're Starting to Feel a Bit Queasy

The term "morning sickness" was probably coined by a man. Perhaps he only saw his wife vomiting on his way to work in the morning and was oblivious to her suffering the rest of the day. —SAMANTHA

Talk about a rude awakening! You're still basking in the new and miraculous knowledge that you're pregnant—dreaming of little booties, and chubby cheeks smeared with strained sweet potatoes—when all of a sudden, you wake up one morning and just the thought of a cup of coffee leaves you feeling clammy and nauseous. Your first thought (poor deluded soul) is that maybe you have the flu. Wrong. Guess what: it's morning sickness, and it's here to stay for a while. It's a queasiness that instead of getting over, you're going to have to get used to.

Now let me say from the outset that morning sickness is

different for every woman. Though it's estimated that any-where from two-thirds to three-fourths of all pregnant women suffer some degree of pregnancy-related nausea or vomiting, no two women I have spoken to shared the exact same experience. *In general*, it strikes at about six or seven weeks, and *in general*, it starts to go away by about week twelve. Some women feel only a persistent but mild queasi-ness. Some women vomit every single day. Some women have to be hospitalized with a serious condition called *Hyperemesis Gravidarum*. And then, curiously enough, some women don't get it at all. Not even a hiccup. We hate them. (Allright, perhaps "envy" would be a more charitable word. But we secretly hope their labor and delivery lasts for days!)

It's estimated that anywhere from ⅔ to ¾ of all pregnant women suffer some degree of pregnancy-related nausea or vomiting; no two women I have spoken to shared the exact same experience. In general, *it strikes at about 6 or 7 weeks, and* in general, *it starts to go away by about week 12.*

The reality is that what we *know* about morning sick-ness pales in comparison to what we *don't know*. In fact, there's so little hard, empirical data on the topic that you might think morning sickness is a medical mystery. There are several reasons for this. First, it's a woman's problem. I don't mean to be cynical here, a basher of the male medical establishment, but even male doctors have told me that if morning sickness happened to men, we'd know a lot more about it by now. Second, studying, researching, and testing pregnant women presents many ethical problems. We can't recreate symptoms of nausea and vomiting in human subjects to see how they work and how to modify them. Third, nausea, like pain, is a highly subjective phenomenon and very difficult to measure in a meaningful way. And fourth, we know that morning sickness most often signifies a viable pregnancy leading to the birth of a healthy baby, so there's little incentive and few research dollars—in a world plagued by cancer, Alzheimer's disease, and AIDS—to study it in depth.

Research has also been hampered by the fact that there is no good animal model to study. Whether you're an animal-rights person or not, the truth is that when it comes to great medical discoveries, some animal in some lab somewhere has made the sacrifice for we humans. But so far, a kindred animal suffering morning sickness has yet to surface. Apes have not provided reliable information when monitored in captivity, because their diets are controlled by people. And according to Jane Goodall—who devoted an entire career to observing chimpanzees, our closest relatives, in the wild—there's little to suggest that pregnant females are ill. There is anecdotal evidence that when domestic dogs become pregnant, their appetites drop significantly around the third week, but this has not been substantiated. We are on our own, at least as a species.

We can take some comfort in knowing that morning sickness is a global phenomenon. Women in unheard-of nomadic tribes and in industrialized superpowers can become members of a new U.N.: that is, United in Nausea. To the !Kung San hunter-gatherers of the Kalahari Desert, the first sign of pregnancy is the onset of vomiting and the unexplained dislike for certain foods. Japanese women suffer the highest reported rates of morning sickness in the world. Though no two women may have the same experience, and it varies from culture to culture and country to country, it is everywhere!

Because of a lack of hard, scientific data, there's plenty of morning-sickness folklore. The first legend, of course, is that crackers make it go away. Another tall tale is that you can determine the sex of your child by the severity of symptoms. Depending on who you talk to, girls cause more trouble than boys. A survey of more than three thou-

A survey of more than 3,000 Swedish women found that those with the most severe form of morning sickness, known as Hyperemesis Gravidarum, had more female infants. There is no study showing a link between male infants and morning sickness.

sand Swedish women found that those with the most severe form of morning sickness, known as *Hyperemesis Gravidarum*, had more *female* infants. There is no study showing a link between male infants and morning sickness. I have one of each and was much sicker with my son.

And, of course, if there's one whopper of an untruth,

Studies show that fewer than 2 percent of women have symptoms only in the morning.

one myth that must be debunked, it is that morning sickness happens in the morning. Nothing could be further from the truth. Studies show that fewer than 2 percent of women have symptoms only in the morning. If you're like me, the late-afternoon into early evening hours are intolerable, making dinnertime an utter chore. Other women feel a gnawing nausea at all hours, to be relieved only by sleep. Morning sickness became known as "morning sickness" because the stomach is emptiest in the morning, when stomach acids are believed to make nausea and queasiness more potent. But in fact, many women report that the symptoms are exacerbated by stress and fatigue, which often make it *worse* later on in the day.

Attempts have been made to give it a new name. Pregnancy sickness is one. Vicki Iovine, in her book *The Girl-*

friend's Guide to Pregnancy, calls it "progesterone poisoning," but it's not really the progesterone that's causing the problems. The medical establishment, never too quick with a catchy phrase for the lay public, has come up with Nausea and Vomiting in Pregnancy, or NVP. A little clinical. Some have suggested pregnancy wellness and pregnancy insurance, since research has now linked morning sickness with a *decreased* risk of miscarriage and with one of the first signs of a healthy pregnancy.

But nothing really sticks like calling it plain old-fashioned morning sickness, so for the purposes of historical continuity and name recognition, I am titling this book *The Morning Sickness Companion*. But let's be clear: it's not happening in the morning, and—perhaps most important—*you're not sick!* In fact, though you may not believe it during these grueling, horrid months of vomiting, strange cravings, and powerful aversions, if there's one thing we do know for sure about morning sickness, it is that it means you are quite well. Your body is functioning beautifully.

2

It's Just Hormones

I was very emotional. Getting stuck in traffic would put me in tears . . . then I'd laugh at how silly I was for crying. I felt all alone at times. —JENNY L.

I don't know about you, but I tend to bristle at the notion that when women are having problems in life, it's always blamed on hormones. It's as if we can't control our emotions and behavior but are slaves to a complex and fickle chemical soup bubbling through our veins, making us crazy or weepy or bitchy or sleepy. Last time I checked, men had endocrine systems, too! But here's one case where hormones *can* take the rap, and I'm okay with it.

We can map the human genome, clone sheep, and send an e-mail to Timbuktu, yet no one knows for certain what causes morning sickness. There are simply too many ethi-

There are more than 30 hormones involved in maintaining a healthy pregnancy.

cal constraints involved in doing research on pregnant women, so in fact, we may *never* know the exact mechanism. But we do know that there are more than thirty hormones involved in maintaining a healthy pregnancy. Among the most notable and notorious: estrogen, progesterone, and HCG (*Human Chorionic Gonadotropin*). HCG, known as "the pregnancy hormone," is the stuff that turns the little pink line in your home-pregnancy test pink and starts to run amok the second an egg is fertilized and implanted in the uterine lining. It is well documented that the early weeks of pregnancy are accompanied by a sharp increase in levels of HCG in the blood, and starting around week twelve, the end of the first trimester, the levels begin to decrease. The spike and subsequent lull of HCG so perfectly parallel most bouts of morning sickness that most doctors believe HCG is the main culprit. Estrogen and progesterone are also highly suspect and responsible for other symptoms: breast tenderness, the one-degree temperature elevation associated with pregnancy, and an increased risk of blood-clot formation, to name a few. As I said, we don't know for a fact that HCG is causing all the nausea and vomiting, and we don't really know how it works, either. Some speculate that HCG upsets the gastrointestinal tract. Others believe the hormones are meddling with the vomiting centers of the brain, or the vestibular canals in the ear that regulate balance and equilibrium. We just don't know, but in this poorly understood phenomenon, hormonal havoc in the name of HCG is the best explanation medicine has to offer.

For years, before the hormonal links emerged, the prevailing wisdom (if you can call it that) was that morning sickness was caused by psychological problems. Women complaining of nausea and vomiting during pregnancy were thought to be either rejecting their pregnancies, rejecting their femininity, depressed about an unplanned pregnancy, too dependent on their mothers (my favorite wacky theory!), or repulsed by the idea of sex, marriage, and childbearing. Believe it or not, these neurosis-based theories remained popular until the mid-twentieth century. Some people still believe it's all in our heads.

Once the *body* became suspect, all kinds of potential

Women complaining of nausea and vomiting during pregnancy were thought to be either rejecting their pregnancies, rejecting their femininity, depressed about an unplanned pregnancy, too dependent on their mothers, or repulsed by the idea of sex, marriage, and childbearing.

causes were floated. There was a belief that morning sickness was the result of problems with the reproductive system such as endometriosis, deep cervical tears, and "incarcerated retroflexed uteruses," which, I guess, had to be freed from jail in order for the symptoms to go away.

So here we are in the twenty-first century, blaming hormones, and of course, the placenta, which excretes them. The problem is that because women differ hormonally and their reactions are so variable, as we've mentioned, no two women will have the same experience; morning sickness is nearly impossible to generalize. No matter how many "books" and "experts" say you should be feeling better right around week twelve, you may not be. In fact, some doctors believe the average time frame for symptoms to go away is more like seventeen to eighteen weeks. Or, if you're one of the unfortunate ones like me, you may feel nauseous and rotten well into your sixth month, and have that awful taste in your mouth right up until the moment your cherub appears. Or maybe you're carrying twins or *more*! Your morning sickness may be doubly bad for twice as long.

What I'm getting at is, *don't* mark the calendar and expect that on the morning of the first day of your thirteenth week, you are going to wake up and want that cappuccino. That's what I did, and it only led to a lot of dashed hopes and unmet expectations: never good things on the best of days, let alone when you are chronically on the verge of vomiting. Let your hormones and your body do their thing, and don't feel bad that you continue to feel bad. It's not unusual.

3

What's Normal?

The emotional toll was overwhelming. I remember attending the first-time parenting class with my husband and ten other couples. I was the only one there who did not enjoy being pregnant, because I was so sick. I thought at least one other first-time mom would empathize with me; certainly I couldn't be the only one. But I was. And that was a very lonely feeling. —ANN F.

Here's another myth about early pregnancy if you're a morning sickness sufferer. You may be perfectly healthy, but *there is no glow.* Glow? I think that if I was ever glowing, it was from the beads of perspiration constantly bursting out on my brow and upper lip as I fretted about where I would be able to puke in public without completely humiliating myself. I was more a shade of dull grayish green those first few weeks. There were days I was so miserable I had to wonder: is it normal to be so sick? Am I hurting the baby with all this nausea and vomiting and the unrelenting craving for Blimpie's turkey subs? The answer is, it *is* normal. And you will *not* hurt the baby by subsisting on cheeseburgers for four months if that's what helps. Morning sickness has, after all, been around for a while. It was described in detail as early as the first century A.D. by a Greek physician, Soranus of Ephesus. He wrote:

> . . . those with this condition are affected with the following: a stomach which is upset, indeed full of fluid; nausea and want of appetite, sometimes for all, sometimes for certain foods. Appetite for things not customary like earth, charcoal, tendrils of the vine, unripe and acid fruit; excessive flow of saliva, malaise, acid eructation, slowness of digestion and a rapid decomposition of food.

Other than wanting to eat earth and charcoal (which some women really do in a rare condition called "pica"), does this sound like you? I find it amazing and quite comforting that as long as two thousand years ago, pregnant women were experiencing the same misery . . . with no ginger ale and crackers to fall back on.

Things haven't changed much. Here is the modern list of basic symptoms you are likely to experience if you have garden-variety morning sickness. You may have some of them, or, God help you, all of them. And remember, they will vary in degrees from woman to woman, so run everything you are feeling by your doctor!

Here is the Modern List of Basic Symptoms:

- *fatigue*

- *nausea or queasiness*

- *vomiting once a day*

- *vomiting several times a day*

- *gag reflexes and dry heaves*

- *powerful food aversions*

- *powerful food cravings*

- *the desire to eat something, only to get it and be nauseated by it*

- *food indecision: a complete inability to decide what you want to eat*

- *overwhelming reactions to smells*

- *bad, funny, or metallic taste in your mouth*

- *overactive salivary glands: a return to the drooling capacity of your teething years*

- *heartburn*

- *acid reflux*

Are we having fun yet?
Abdominal pain and tenderness, fever, and headache

are not considered typical symptoms of morning sickness, and if you are experiencing these things, you should see your doctor.

Hyperemesis

If are you vomiting all day long and unable to keep *any* food down, you may have a condition called *Hyperemesis Gravidarum*: an extreme form of morning sickness that afflicts about 1 percent of pregnant women. THIS IS NOT NORMAL OR HEALTHY, AND YOU SHOULD SEE YOUR DOCTOR RIGHT AWAY. How do you know if you have hyperemesis and not an average case of morning sickness? Other than the obvious inability to keep any food or liquid down, the first measurable sign of a serious problem is *weight loss* of greater than 5 percent of your pre-pregnancy weight. Pregnant women should always be steadily gaining weight, not losing it. Also, your doctor should do tests to see if there are ketones in your urine. Excessive ketones in the urine (known as ketonuria) are a sign that the body is not using carbohydrates from food for

Hyperemesis Gravidarum: an extreme form of morning sickness that afflicts about 1 percent of pregnant women.

fuel and instead, is trying to break down fat for fuel. Ketonuria is often the first physical symptom of starvation.

Left untreated, hyperemesis can lead to dehydration, electrolyte imbalances, neurologic problems, liver and kidney damage, and yes, even death for the mother, although that is *very rare* in this day and age. In the old days, not only did women die during childbirth, but many died as a result of hyperemesis as well. Charlotte Brontë, the British author of *Jane Eyre*, is said to have died of hyperemesis. And although hyperemesis has been associated with an increased risk of fetal loss and low birth weight, it is generally considerred more of a risk to the mother than to the unborn baby.

No one is quite sure what causes hyperemesis. Some believe that if morning sickness were graded on a bell curve, the women with hyperemesis would simply represent the worst possible cases. It is seen more often in first pregnancies and in pregnancies of multiple babies, i.e., twins and triplets. Because it can be very serious, hospitalization and intravenous hydration are often necessary, but several doctors with whom I have spoken assure me that the condition is easily recognized and that treatment is available and effective. There are drugs on the market that can control the vomiting and are considered safe for the baby. (More on that in the chapter on treatment.) I want to emphasize that most of the information in this book may not apply to women with hyperemesis. I am trying to provide tools for managing the average case of morning sickness, but the most severe cases will need constant medical intervention.

You should also check with your doctor if your morning sickness persists well beyond the fourteen- to seventeen-week range. Longer-term nausea may be the result of thyroid abnormalities. An overactive or an underactive thyroid could be a problem for mother and baby and should be corrected. And in rare cases, liver disease may be the source of symptoms, so a set of liver-function tests may be necessary for women with nausea that just won't quit after the fourteenth week.

4

It's Not Just Nausea

For me, it was definitely a time of depression, and to be honest, anger. I hated how I felt, hated how I looked, how endless the whole thing seemed. Each day dragged by and I was counting off each one. ——MARY JANE C.

There's one more symptom of morning sickness that I think is so important and so under-discussed that I want to give it its own chapter, and that is depression. I'm using the word loosely here because it could be a mild but persistent case of the blues stemming from how dismayed you feel about yourself, or it could be a full-blown clinical depression requiring that you get some help. Either way, there is no denying that morning sickness takes an enormous psychological and emotional toll and greatly affects the quality of life of women who go through it. They often report feeling isolated, angry, betrayed by their bodies and babies, and misunderstood. They don't sleep well, don't work well, can't concentrate, and develop strained relationships with their partners, families, and employers. In the limited scientific research available on the topic, a survey of 3,201 pregnant women in Canada and the United States found that 20 percent of women with "mild" morning sickness reported feeling depressed most of the time. Thirty percent of women with moderate symptoms were frequently depressed, and for those with severe symptoms, 50 percent said they were always depressed.

And yet I am utterly astonished to find almost nothing written about the "trauma" of morning sickness in the vast selection of pregnancy books on bookstore shelves. In most discussions, morning sickness is given short shrift anyway, but even in those books that devote a page or two to the topic, no one says: "PS: Not only might you be feeling nauseous for three months, but working, taking care of another child, being a good spouse, and just being yourself might also be *monumental challenges!*"

Dr. Gideon Koren, who runs the organization "Motherisk," calls the issue of emotional and psychological problems stemming from morning sickness a "black hole." Little research is being done. Few people are interested in studying it, and as a result, next to nothing is known, written, or discussed about something very real and potentially devastating to women. And it's not just women with the most severe type of morning sickness, known as hyperemesis, but women with even mild to moderate symptoms who also must find a way to get on with their lives.

∽

A survey of 3,201 pregnant women in Canada and the United States found that 20 percent of women with "mild" morning sickness reported feeling depressed most of the time. Thirty percent of women with moderate symptoms were frequently depressed, and for those with severe symptoms, 50 percent said they were always depressed.

If I didn't know that I was pregnant, I would have thought that I was terminally ill. Between being constantly tired and sluggish, feeling nauseated and unable to keep food down, I was very debilitated.

—RUTH K.

I kept looking through book after book hoping to find some validation of my own feelings and came away wondering if there was something wrong with me that I was so dispirited, disheveled, and dismayed.

Why is that? My guess is that for much of the world, depression really is still a stigma, and since morning sickness is temporary and is *generally* associated with a healthy outcome, perhaps there's a sense that in this case, it's not worth talking about. We should just be tough and get over it. And above all, we're supposed to feel unfettered joy about being pregnant, not sadness and ambivalence. This may be one of the hardest incongruities to wrestle with during morning sickness. In reality, we know we are blessed to be pregnant, but it can be next to impossible to feel gratitude for our fecundity when we are puking in the aisle at Kmart.

There were times I would break down after vomiting excessively. I would kneel in front of a bucket and cry aloud. I would say things like "Why doesn't this baby like me?" "Why is he/she doing this to me?" And "I hate being pregnant. I never want another kid.

—ANATILDE G.

When I knew I was pregnant with my second child, my first reaction was one of overwhelming dread (something I didn't feel I could discuss with my husband or friends) and it was directly related to having to face another round of morning sickness. I felt incredibly selfish in a way.

—CHRIS H.

There are rare cases of women who choose to terminate pregnancies because of morning sickness, *many* cases of women who contemplate doing so, and even more cases of women who resent being pregnant in general because it takes such a physical toll. These feelings are common, but are worth taking up with your doctor if you can't escape them.

> *I hated myself, hated myself for not being able to bear the whole thing better. This was supposed to be the most joyous experience. I wanted to have children very much. Having heard of so many people with fertility problems, I knew that I was blessed to even become pregnant. But I was miserable. I wanted to suck it up courageously, but I didn't. I just got through it with lots of crying, moaning, and complaining. Not exactly my finest moments.* —MARY JANE C.

> *I did not want to go out of the house. I felt . . . nauseous. People would call me to congratulate me and all I felt was ill, and like I wanted to curl up into the shape of the new fetus.* —MARY G.

The depression element of morning sickness may give credence to that old-fashioned theory that it's all in our heads, but the more modern understanding is that depression is the result of the nausea and vomiting rather than depression or neurosis causing nausea and vomiting. It's hard *not* to feel bad when you're chronically, if temporarily, ill and the whole world is telling you to be happy.

I felt weak, and I felt as though I would need a lot of medical help during pregnancy and birth. So mentally I felt weakened, and therefore, decisions I made about how to handle the birthing process later down the line were influenced. After the morning sickness ended and I felt strong again, I completely reversed the decisions I had made about my doctor and hospital while under the weakening influence of morning sickness. I think that's very much something for women to be aware of . . . that change of heart after the morning sickness has lifted. —ANONYMOUS

The nausea in my pregnancy contributed to the profoundly disorienting experience of not feeling like myself. I just wanted to escape through sleep. No other conscious experience would alleviate the misery except the actual act of eating. While chewing and ingesting food, I didn't feel so aware of the nausea, so I ate constantly and gained 50 to 55 pounds in my first two pregnancies and I am sure I am headed for 60 this time no doubt. This was terribly discouraging and depressing for me as a normally fit and active person. I felt so out of control. —CHRIS S.

Yes, morning sickness involves an almost total loss of control. Women who are used to feeling healthy and strong all of a sudden perceive themselves as weak and vulnerable. Simple tasks require Herculean effort. An estimated 25 percent of nauseous pregnant women require time off from their jobs because they feel so sick. The daily pleasure of eating becomes a chore. The joy of expectant motherhood is a casualty in the never-ending battle to get through the day.

> . . . It was unbelievable. First of all, very few people understand what you are going through. Second, I had this expectation that pregnancy was going to feel great and was terribly disappointed that instead of glowing, I spent most of my time wanting to die. Being nauseated for nine months was an experience that shook me to my bones. I have had to deal with serious pain before and coped really well with it . . . but nausea is a feeling there is nowhere to escape, no way to take your mind off it. —KERRY M.

An estimated 25 percent of nauseous pregnant women require time off from their jobs because they feel so sick.

> Being sick made me feel horrible. I couldn't go to restaurants I liked. I couldn't go to parties because I was afraid I would embarrass myself if I threw up at the wrong moment. If I got into a car, there

would be a bucket in case I vomited. Vomiting made
my whole body hurt from the inside out.
                                                —ANATILDE G.

Complicating matters, conventional wisdom tells us we should not tell people we are pregnant until *after* the first trimester, when many cases of morning sickness have already run their course. That means that you have to suffer in silence when you are at your sickest: a lonely predicament.

I looked sick and pale all the time, besides getting big.
It was hard not to tell people about my pregnancy (I
don't like to tell before three months), so I basically
stopped socializing for three months.   —KYOKO H.

Unfortunately, all the books and general opinion say
that you should not tell anyone until the third or fourth
month. This meant that at a period when I was most
in need of sisterhood about this condition, there was no
one to talk to about it.   —PAXTON B.

My suggestion is to defy books and general opinion and find a confidante or two. I was so sick and unable to function that I felt I had to tell my boss when I was only about nine or ten weeks pregnant, because I thought he deserved an explanation for why I was suddenly missing in action. And you know what? He was incredibly decent and understanding about the whole thing. Only you can judge how people will respond. And look at it this way: if, God forbid, your pregnancy doesn't work out and you miscarry, you'll want to talk to people about that experience anyway.

For me, there were two major hurdles each and every day—how to do my job, and how to care for my energetic three-year-old daughter. Both required me to move slowly, to be creative, and to be forgiving of myself. I had trouble concentrating, talking to people, and working under pressure, but at the office, at least I could vomit in peace and then lie down on a couch. I didn't exactly feel like Employee of the Month, but one thing that really helped was talking about it. Early on in my pregnancy, I confided in my producer and good friend Susan Schiller that I was suffering terrible morning sickness. Having been through it herself, she understood and picked up the slack for me. I realize that not all of you will have the luxury of working with or for sympathetic women, but this underscores my point that at least confiding in someone takes a little of the pressure off.

In general, I believe that people will be understanding and excited for you that you are pregnant, a happiness you may well have forgotten and could stand to be reminded of from time to time as you cope with feeling so sick.

Working actually seemed to help as it would/could divert my attention from the nausea and thus lessen its effects a wee bit. —HEATHER S.

Many women I have interviewed have echoed that sentiment and have told me they found work to be a positive distraction, and that morning-sickness symptoms became more pronounced when they had more time to dwell on how they were feeling. So don't quit your day job! Working can help you keep your mind off things and remind you that you're capable and strong and can get through it.

I built in the time it took to get sick into my schedule, so I got up earlier to get sick and then get to work on time. —PAT L.

Don't quit your day job! Working can help you keep your mind off things and remind you that you're capable and strong and can get through it.

It would take me one and a half to two hours to get ready for work. I would shower, lay down for 15 minutes, get up, dry my hair and lay down for 15 minutes and so on, until I was ready to leave."   —ELLA D.

I'm a middle-school teacher, so I'm around kids all day long. Sometimes I would have to eat during class, which was distracting to my students, or I would feel drained from throwing up or feeling nauseous all the time, so I was often lethargic during class or distracted.
—NICKY R.

It only affected my work in that I had to have food constantly available and had to stay near a bathroom.
—CATHY C.

There were days I was unable to get out of bed because movement made me sick, certain smells made me sick . . . cigarette smoke was the worst smell of them all. So therfor [sic] I was fired from my job 'cause I was unable to get up to go every day."   —LYNNETTE F.

It was very difficult to come home from work and take care of my three-and-a-half-year-old. I would kind of curl up on the couch and we'd eat crackers together.
—SUSAN S.

And that leads me to my next topic: caring for the kids. You can confide in them, too, saying: "Mommy doesn't feel well today," and they will look at you with those big eyes, half concerned, half suspicious, and say, "That's too bad, Mommy. Now can we play monster? You're the monster who chases me."

I didn't want to play, my level of patience was at an all-time low, I had trouble preparing meals, and basically, I didn't want to do anything but watch videos. Like it or not, the television could become your new best friend, and you have to let that be okay for a few months. When we did go to the playground, I would sit on a bench in as much shade as I could find and eat all the crackers and snacks I had brought for my daughter. Luckily, at three, my daughter was old enough to be out of diapers, as I am told that changing diapers when suffering from morning sickness can be a traumatic experience

> *I was depressed that I couldn't be energetic for my son and felt extremely guilty that I didn't want to play with him. I just wanted to lay down, especially after not seeing him all day.* —JUNE N.

In general, women with morning sickness feel a lot of guilt about their inability to care for a small child, and concern as their young ones watch them get sick. Children tend to be fascinated with throwing up and will ask a lot of questions. If they happen to catch you in the act, just be honest about what is happening, let them help as much as you can tolerate, and reassure them that you will eventually be okay.

Which, of course, you will.

I would throw up at home and my two-year-old son started caressing the toilet bowl and making retching noises! Just like Mommy!   —RUTH K.

I was extremely nauseous and fatigued and it greatly affected our family life. I would fall asleep on the couch every afternoon while my three- and five-year-olds watched Barney.   —CHRIS H.

Very challenging to prepare meals for my toddler when the sight and smell of food is so nauseating . . . hard to climb monkey bars or push him in the swings, too.

—LU H.

The second pregnancy, my first son was two and very demanding. I had to lie on his floor and try to get him to play by himself.   —LOUISA W.

My second baby was born 13 months after my first, so luckily I just snuggled up with him. While pregnant with my third, I would drive one to nursery school, rush back to nap the second, and lie half-sleeping in a queasy nauseous sweat until 3:00 P.M.

—CHRISTINE K.

To this day, when I hear the "music" to Nintendo Super Mario, it makes me somewhat sick. The reason is because I was so nauseous I would let the kids play Nintendo all morning long.   —LORI S.

I was rendered incompetent roughly half the time. I vividly remember my first child watching me retch with a combination of fascination and horror on his face. The whole thing was really vile.   —KERRY M.

It was draining and a struggle. Sometimes when I felt like I could not eat or I would throw up, I would feel guilty and ashamed . . . like I'm already a bad mom.
                                                —NICKY R.

And finally, there's one other element of morning sickness that can make life extremely grim for several months: not only do we feel like hell, we often *look* like hell, too. Let's face it, women are vain creatures at heart. We want to look our best just like anybody else, but vomiting every day combined with gorging ourselves on grilled cheese can lead to a woman's worst nightmare: feeling *fat* and *ugly*. Of course I am not saying that you *are*, but it's the perception that counts, and we are always our harshest critics.

Whenever I threw up, I broke dozens of tiny blood vessels under my eyes and on my nose. I found that simple efforts to make myself look better, like taking a shower and holding a hair dryer up to my head, were exhausting, and of course none of my clothes fit right anymore, getting tighter and tighter by the day. On top of that, I had to spend my day on-camera. I was dying a slow death. I owe a debt of gratitude to Dan Rather, who used to poke his head in my office routinely and tell me I had a primordial (his word) beauty when I was pregnant. I would do one of those double takes, looking over my shoulder to see if he was talking to someone else. I think one day I even told him he needed glasses. But the bottom line is that Dan will never know how much that meant to me at such a low point in my life.

I felt everything about my appearance kind of droop. My skin, my hair, my clothes just didn't look right. The amazing thing was that I just didn't care very much. —LAURA P.

Physically, I always looked good. I enjoyed buying maternity clothes, doing my hair, etc. My motto: I felt like shit, but man, I was gonna look good! That probably got me through those awful times. —LORI S.

I never swelled up but my face was drained of all its color. I avoided mirrors and people. I disliked everyone around me who was having a better pregnancy. —ANATILDE G.

Here are some suggestions. Be very forgiving of yourself at this time. So you're not the glamour queen you usually are; it's hard work making a baby! Find a few simple pieces of clothing that work and are comfortable, and don't obsess about fashion. Cut your hair in a simple style that is easy to care for. Buy a new shade of lipstick. Get regular manicures and pedicures. Do the little things that make you feel well-groomed and better about yourself. Remember that soon you'll feel beautiful again *and* you'll have a beautiful baby on your hip to boot.

We've addressed a lot of the emotional and psychological battles women with morning sickness must fight every day. Some are easier to deal with than others, and some we *can* laugh about. But I can't stress enough the importance of talking to your doctor if you are extremely depressed. Don't downplay your feelings. Morning sickness is *not* just a physical malady: it's draining, stressful, and exhausting. It will color every aspect of your life for its duration. Luckily, it's temporary.

Find a few simple pieces of clothing that work and are comfortable, and don't obsess about fashion. Cut your hair in a simple style that is easy to care for. Buy a new shade of lipstick. Get regular manicures and pedicures. Do the little things that make you feel well-groomed and better about yourself. Remember that soon you'll feel beautiful again and you'll have a beautiful baby on your hip to boot.

5

The Nose Knows

Odors bothered me most. I changed every scent in my house. I bought unscented bar soap, deodorant, detergent. I could smell a fire in the next town.

—ELIZABETH P. G.

Perhaps one of the most curious symptoms of morning sickness is something called "hyperolfaction," an extremely heightened sense of smell. You become like a dog tuning in to a high-pitched whistle, or—a more accurate canine comparison—a bloodhound picking up a remote scent. The mildest aromas assault you. Smells you once loved, like bacon cooking or your husband's aftershave lotion, become unbearable.

That after-dinner drink and his cologne had to go!

—HILARY T.

No one is quite sure why this happens, but there are some theories claiming that estrogen somehow enhances the sense of smell. This is a helpful tidbit of information when you are working on avoiding the things that make you sick. In her book *No More Morning Sickness*, dietician Miriam Erick writes: "My practice has convinced me that most of the physical complaints of morning sickness begin with the nose."

This is an important point. Many bouts of nausea related to food are triggered by smells. The aroma of cooking food, and especially of meat, can be one of the most noxious things a woman with morning sickness can encounter. Since we all have to breathe, the only remedy for this side effect is avoidance. Be sure to ventilate your home, get fresh air, and give up cooking if you can.

> *Oddly enough, the one time I was less plagued by nausea was during my first and third pregnancies when I developed sinus infections and could not breathe at all through my nose. As soon as my infections lifted, my symptoms returned in full force.* —CHRIS SIEVE

Of course, few women can really "give up" cooking, especially if their husbands or partners are culinarily challenged. Thankfully, that is less of an issue in this modern era than it used to be, and even men who consider a kitchen a foreign land can boil water to make pasta, put together a

Many bouts of nausea related to food are triggered by smells. The aroma of cooking food, and especially of meat, can be one of the most noxious things a woman with morning sickness can encounter.

grilled-cheese sandwich or, if push comes to shove, order take-out. So if odors are really your trigger, you might have to give up the serious cooking for a while and delegate. Stock your kitchen with things that are easy to prepare and not too redolent: pasta, baked potatoes, canned soups, yogurt, fruit, et cetera.

Prepared frozen foods are not terribly good for you and are loaded with sodium, but during this temporary struggle with morning sickness, they are fair game. In the sur-

Stock your kitchen with things that are easy to prepare and not too redolent: like pasta, baked potatoes, canned soups, yogurt, fruit, et cetera.

veys, one woman said she lived on Stouffer's Turkey Tetrazzini, and I've already mentioned my sister-in-law Chris, who got through every morning with the help of Lean Cuisine. She wouldn't consider frozen dinners post-pregnancy, but at the time, they saved her. Wouldn't it be great if the frozen-food manufacturers could come up with a product just for women with morning sickness? Then we'd have both Hungry Man and Nauseous Woman dinners on the market! But seriously, frozen foods are simply too convenient not to consider, and one of the best things about them is that they don't smell!

Another thing you might want to try is to set up an "odor-free" zone in your home, a little sanctuary where you can be protected from offending smells when you are feelings nauseous. Keep the doors closed, don't allow the pets in, and filter out any strong smells from the outside world. There is a whole range of unscented products on the market to help you do this. Wash your clothes, sheets, pillowcases, and towels in unscented detergents. Buy unscented bath soap and deodorant. Check your local health-food

Wash your clothes, sheets, pillowcases, and towels in unscented detergents. Buy unscented bath soap and deodorant. Check your local health-food store for fragrance-free shampoo, or try something, very mild like baby shampoo.

store for frangrance-free shampoo, or try something very mild like baby shampoo. You might also want to invest in a fan or an air filter just to keep a nice breeze blowing. If certain fragrances are soothing to you (lavender or citrus were two that I found tolerable), you can try masking other offending odors in your house with scented candles that you like, or air-fresheners that claim to wick bad smells away. A word of caution, though: nothing smells worse than a bad smell being drowned out by a supposedly nice smell. Use anything fragranced sparingly. I think neutral smells are your best bet.

Of course, you can't hide in your odor-free zone for several months. There will be days when you will be on that stuffy, crowded bus next to a woman who has doused herself in an entire bottle of Eau de Puke, or maybe you will have to walk by an outside food cart reeking of onions and peppers on your way to work in the morning. For these uncomfortable moments, I have one suggestion. It may sound silly, but sometimes there's nothing quite as effective as breathing through your mouth!

There's not much more to say on the subject except, well, morning sickness stinks!

6

What Would Darwin Say?

Each day I would wake up and worry. How bad is it going to be today?
                                                    —EVA L.

If you're kneeling over that toilet bowl or sink every day crying out why, Why, WHY? there may be an answer for you, or at least an intriguing evolutionary theory to ponder. It might succeed in taking your mind off your suffering for a while. Could it be possible that the reason some women vomit and are drawn to some foods while being literally nauseated by others is *not* just a random act of torture designed to make us never have more than one child, but instead, a carefully orchestrated phenomenon that has helped us protect our unborn babies over millions of years of evolution?

The theory has been put forth by several scientists,

most notably the evolutionary biologist Margie Profet, who has written extensively on the topic. She argues that human pregnancy sickness evolved over the ages as a way to shield the developing baby from any food that could be considered a "teratogen," a term you'll come across frequently if you read much science about pregnancy. It means anything causing birth defects. For our ancestors, that might have meant plants, herbs, and spices that contained natural toxins called phytochemicals, or meats that had spoiled.

For modern women, it could be alcohol and caffeine. Have you ever noticed that most women who love their evening glass of red wine will eagerly avoid it once in the throes of morning sickness? Many find giving up alcohol in the first trimester is one of the easiest sacrifices to make because they simply lose all taste for it. Is it because all of a sudden they hate red wine? Or because the wine poses a threat to the developing embryo? Since we know that alcohol is in fact a teratogen, the theory is that perhaps it isn't coincidental that we want to avoid it during those first delicate weeks of pregnancy.

But there are other less obvious examples. Many pregnant women with morning sickness have powerful aversions to the stronger-tasting vegetables; spinach and broccoli can lose all appeal, for example. Is there something about those foods that could have posed a potential threat in bygone days? Profet would say yes. She believes that because natural toxins exist in most plants, humans developed strong aversions to them, even to the point of throwing them up to protect the fetus.

Because the human body cannot possibly know inherently which particular toxins, of the vast spectrum that exist in nature, would cause defects in the embryo's organ formation, pregnancy sickness is designed to recognize general cues of toxicity . . . pungent odors and bitter tastes are the main cues of toxins. Pregnancy sickness causes the woman to have strong aversions to these cues. Even a woman's most cherished foods can become unpalatable or nauseating. (Profet, *Pregnancy Sickness*, p. 6)

It does make sense when you think about foods that appeal to most women suffering morning sickness: bland foods, breads and crackers, fruit, nothing too spicy. I defy you to show me the woman with morning sickness who craves a serving of kale and then washes it down with a strong cup of coffee. Technically, kale and coffee in moderation are *not* teratogens, but they are strong, bitter-tasting plants containing phytochemicals. Maybe our ancestors thought they were just better off avoiding them.

To test Profet's theory, two evolutionary biologists at Cornell University also investigated the matter. Professor Paul Sherman and graduate student Sam Flaxman looked up every single study they could find on the frequency of morning sickness and came up with fifty-six, analyzing a total of seventy-nine thousand pregnancies. The first thing they learned from all those studies was that two-thirds to three-fourths of pregnant women worldwide experienced some degree of morning sickness. Their first conclusion then was that morning sickness was simply too common to be something that is *bad*. Over all evolutionary time, if it was really causing harm, if it was really a defect or disease, we as a species would have gotten rid of it in order to survive. And yet it persists from woman to woman, country to country, culture to culture. Hmmmm. The logical deduction is that this dreadful, unrelenting nausea you are now feeling must have some useful function in the big picture. You are doing yeoman's work for the human race. Feel better? Using a graph (Figure A) to back up their case, Sherman and Flaxman argue that if morning sickness plays a role in protecting the fetus, it should occur at a time in pregnancy when the need for protection is the greatest. If you notice, the embryo is doing its most intricate developing and is most sensitive to damage during those crucial first twelve weeks. Is it coincidental that *most* nausea and

Two-thirds to three-fourths of pregnant women worldwide experience some degree of morning sickness. Over all evolutionary time, if it was really causing harm, if it was really a defect or disease, we as a species would have gotten rid of it in order to survive.

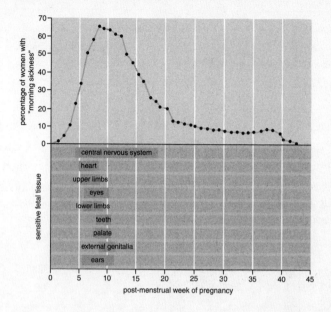

Figure A. Nausea and vomiting tend to peak between the eighth and twelfth weeks of pregnancy, which coincides with the peak sensitivity of various fetal tissues to a chemical disturbance. Emma Skurnick/*American Scientist*

vomiting take place during the first twelve weeks? The evolutionary theorists believe the evidence is simply too strong to be random.

And one other thing: if you take a look at the relationship between the nausea and vomiting of pregnancy and miscarriage in Figure B, you can see that in every study that Sherman and Flaxman could find, there is a lower incidence of miscarriage when there is more nausea and vomiting.

Sherman and Flaxman also analyzed the diets of women with morning sickness and found some interesting correlations with Profet's theory. If you look at Figure C,

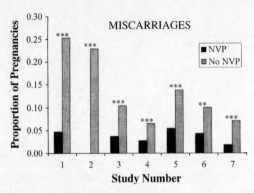

Figure B. Association of NVP with reduced miscarriage rates (fetal death at ≤20 weeks). Paul Sherman and Sam Flaxman

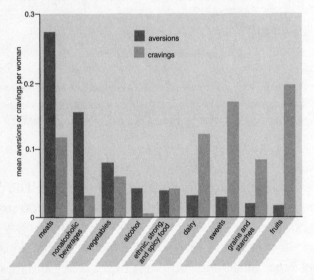

Figure C. Food aversions during pregnancy are more common than cravings for items that might contain harmful toxins, chemicals, or bacteria such as meat (including fish, poultry, and eggs), nonalcoholic beverages (coffee, tea, and sodas, which often contain caffeine), vegetables (which contain phytotoxins), and alcohol. Foods that are craved more than they are found aversive—such as fruits (and fruit juices), grains (breads), sweets (desserts and chocolate), and dairy (including ice cream)—are less likely to contain harmful elements. Emma Skurnick/*American Scientist*

There is a lower incidence of miscarriage when there is more nausea and vomiting.

you can see that the foods pregnant women had strong aversions to included meats, non-alcoholic caffeinated beverages, vegetables, and alcohol—in other words, foods likely to contain toxins or bacteria that could harm the developing embryo. Foods the pregnant women craved included fruits, grains, sweets, and dairy products that would be less likely to be teratogenic. According to Sherman and Flaxman, the strong aversions to meats can be explained by the fact that prior to widespread electric refrigeration, these foods would be most likely to contain bacteria and viruses. Infections during pregnancy can be extremely dangerous to a developing embryo and its mother. There are seven cultures with no morning sickness at all, and studies found these had corn-based diets, while the country with the highest rate of morning sickness was Japan, which bases its diet on fish and shellfish, which can carry a lot of bacteria.

This evolutionary theory raises an important question: something else to think about before you beg your doctor to do anything, Anything, ANYTHING to make it go away. If morning sickness plays a vital role in protecting the developing baby, *should* we attempt to eliminate the dreadful symptoms? After all, the nausea and vomiting and

Studies found there are seven cultures with no morning sickness at all, and these had corn-based diets, while the country with the highest rate of morning sickness was Japan, which bases its diet on fish and shellfish, which can carry a lot of bacteria.

misery are supposedly good for the baby, keeping us away from plant toxins, rancid meats, coffee, and alcohol, right? We may live in the age of refrigeration, preservatives, genetic engineering, and special soaps to rid our foods of pesticides, but food-borne illnesses still afflict an estimated eighty million people a year. One in ten Americans experience bacterial food-poisoning every year. So perhaps your nausea, urging you to run from that salad bar, may actually be the modern-day equivalent of not eating a certain bark or berry that could make you sick. If we eliminate the symptoms, would we wind up eating all sorts of things that could make us and our babies sick?

What about all those women who never have one day of morning sickness? They usually have perfectly healthy, beautiful babies anyway. Are they just statistical anomalies? It's food for thought.

There are some doctors and sufferers of morning sickness who may disagree with the evolutionary theory. Some believe that in the modern age, when the food supply is as clean as it has ever been and 75 percent of women are now in the workforce, perhaps morning sickness is nothing more than an annoyance that has outlived any evolutionary usefulness. Because it can be debilitating, leaving some women unable to perform their jobs or take care of their other youngsters, perhaps it is *not* helping protect the embryo, but is actually interfering with our lives and serves no function whatsoever. And holes in the theory emerge when you consider that many of the foods we have aversions to during morning sickness are technically *not* teratogenic. Broccoli, at least today, doesn't cause birth defects. Neither does spaghetti with tomato sauce, yet I was unable to look at those foods during my first trimester.

Do we really need morning sickness anymore? Personally, I like the evolutionary theory, if for no other reason than it makes me feel I haven't suffered in vain. There's something so miraculous and overwhelming about creating human life—all those little fingers and toes, and perfect little cells dividing and doing exactly what they are meant to do—that I'm thrilled just to believe that my not being able to eat salad for months played a part. I simply can't believe that so many women can be made so miserable for no reason at all. For lack of a better explanation for why morning sickness afflicts so many, perhaps we can find answers and, more important, comfort, in continuity. We have experienced the aversions of the ancestors, and have lived to tell the tale.

7

So What's a Nauseous Girl to Do? The Treatment Dilemma

There's a short version of this chapter . . . and a long one. The short version is this: there is no "medical" treatment for morning sickness except for swallowing a dose of the old adage: "Grin and bear it." Though symptoms have been recorded throughout history and across cultures, not one tried-and-true remedy stands out as consistently relieving discomfort. In addition, few women when pressed really want to take unnecessary medication while they are pregnant. Unless a pregnancy involves the extreme morning sickness known as *Hyperemesis Gravidarum*, many believe there is no medical need to make the symptoms go away. You may be miserable and *want* to die, but neither you nor the baby are in any danger of that. In fact, as we've already discussed in the previous chapter on evolution, some believe there's a benefit to being nauseous and staying nauseous.

Though symptoms have been recorded throughout history and across cultures, not one tried-and-true remedy stands out as consistently relieving discomfort.

Here's the long version. Since the days of Hippocrates in 400 B.C., doctors have been struggling to treat the nausea and vomiting, food aversions and cravings, that come hand in hand with pregnancy. Some of the earliest attempts on record can be found in the writing of Soranus of Ephesus:

At the first sensation, one must fast for one day so that the stomach, not being set in motion as is natural, may be kept undisturbed through rest.

Fast? That would be a tall order. Today we understand that food in the stomach is a better idea for keeping nausea at bay.

After the fast, Soranus prescribes:

> . . . a rubdown with ointment . . . little and easily digested food like a soft-boiled egg or a porridge, and some not very fat fowl as well as water to drink . . .

> . . . and then, finally, a massage:

> After the first days, the woman should take a comparatively hot bath, a little weak wine, and passive exercise . . . she also ought to promenade, exercise the voice, and read aloud with modulations, take active exercise in the form of dancing, punching the leather bag, playing with the ball and by means of massage.

I especially love the "punch the leather bag" treatment. I know there were days I certainly felt like punching *any-*

thing, but that was out of anger and frustration, not nausea.

On a serious note, the recommendations to exercise are valid and well worth heeding. You may feel like never crawling out of bed, but I can say from experience, exercise was one of the few remedies that actually helped. For some reason, during that one-hour prenatal workout class, the motion, music, mirrors, and the company of other waddling women succeeded in taking my mind off my troubles. Something about the physical exertion kept my nausea at bay and I felt alive again. For more on how exercise can help, see chapter 9.

Finally, for women who are really suffering, Soranus advised that the abdomen should be bound with "oil of roses, quinces, myrtle, mastich, spikenard . . ."

And if that doesn't work and nausea persists, he suggests that "It would be advisable to bind the extremities, for by their constriction, the stomach is also affected, or to immerse them in hot water."

After considering these ancient remedies, it would seem we've come a long way, baby. Or have we? Soranus's Rx may sound a little extreme, but believe it or not, in two thousand years, women with morning sickness haven't had many more options. In the late 1700s, doctors tried bleeding and stool softeners since morning sickness was attributed to bloated blood vessels. Then came leeches, opium, and in the nineteenth century, forced dilation of the cervix, which was thought to stop vomiting.

And then came thalidomide. You've probably heard of it because of its prominent place in the annals of medical disasters.

Thalidomide

Thalidomide was first introduced in 1957 in West Germany. It was initially used as a sleeping pill but was eventually found to offer great relief to women suffering morning sickness and became the drug of choice for pregnant women throughout Europe and Canada, Asia, Australia, and Africa.

The German drug company, Chemie Grunenthal, promoted thalidomide as being completely nontoxic and safe for pregnant women, but it turned out that animal tests were never done to measure the effects of the drug on a fetus.

Then, in December 1956, the first of what would be more than ten thousand "thalidomide babies" were born. The infant was the daughter of a Chemie Grunenthal employee who, months before the drug was available to the public, had been bringing samples of it home to soothe his pregnant wife. The little girl was born without ears, but at the time no one made a connection between the thalidomide and the one unfortunate case. What would follow, however, was an epidemic of birth defects linked to thalidomide. Though they spanned several continents, the babies shared similar deformities, most notably "phocomelia," derived from the Greek words "seal" and "limb." Hands and feet were directly attached to the trunk, shoulder, or hip, giving the appearance of "flippers." Forty percent never lived beyond age one, but an estimated five thousand are still alive today. Only after thousands of women took the drug was it discovered that even a single dose could wreak havoc on a developing fetus in the first trimester.

By 1961, before it ever made its way to the United

States, thalidomide was yanked off the market. It left behind a generation of crippled children, and one other less visible legacy: from that point on, all efforts to treat morning sickness pharmaceutically came to a screeching halt. Some doctors call thalidomide the "sentinel event" in the development of drugs for pregnant women, adding that for better or worse, it spawned a culture of hysteria about taking medication while pregnant.

Bendectin

Bendectin may the best-known (pharmaceutical) victim of the thalidomide legacy. First marketed in the United States in 1956, it was widely prescribed by doctors to treat nausea and vomiting in pregnancy and remains the only drug ever approved by the Food and Drug Administration to treat morning sickness. It is estimated that it was used in thirty-three million pregnancies before an avalanche of lawsuits forced its manufacturer, Merrell Dow, voluntarily to pull it off the market in 1983 or be put out of business by mounting legal costs.

What happened was that a number of women came forward claiming that the Bendectin they had taken was responsible for birth defects in their children. Limb deformities, cleft palates, cleft lips, heart disease, and something called "pyloric stenosis"—a malformation of the digestive tract—were blamed on the drug. But definitive scientific evidence linking Bendectin with birth defects was never produced. In fact, more than thirty published studies

Some doctors call thalidomide the "sentinel event" in the development of drugs for pregnant women, adding that for better or worse, it spawned a culture of hysteria about taking medication while pregnant.

involving more than 130,000 patients found no measurable increase in birth defects among those who had used the drug. In 1995, Dr. Robert L. Brent analyzed *all* the available medical literature on Bendectin—two hundred studies, both animal and human—and concluded:

> The epidemiologic and experimental data indicate that the clinical use of Bendectin does not increase the risk of birth defects in populations of exposed pregnant women.

Did women who took Bendectin have babies with birth defects? Yes. Was the Bendectin to blame? Experts say to look at the odds. If you have a baby, there's a 2- to 3-percent chance of birth defects *in general*, so in a population of thirty-three million women, bad luck and Bendectin were

If you have a baby, there's a 2- to 3-percent chance of birth defects in general.

bound to collide. But that fact could not stop the rising tide of lawsuits or prevent the demise of a drug that many doctors say was really harmless and extremely helpful.

The Bendectin case is worth knowing about for several reasons. First of all, it set a legal precedent, becoming the poster child for something we now call "junk science"— science introduced into a court of law unaccompanied by any empirical scientific evidence to back up its claim. Lawyers representing parents who claimed that Bendectin had caused their children's birth defects found and *paid* eight witnesses willing to testify that Bendectin might have been the cause. The case eventually wound up before the United States Supreme Court in 1993, and the court ruled that "expert" testimony on scientific matters had to be carefully screened by judges so as not to confuse jurors. In his book *Voodoo Science*, which discusses the case, Robert Park writes that the high Court ruling noted that:

. . . allowing evidence to be introduced that is not generally accepted by the scientific community would result in a free-for-all in which juries would be confounded by absurd and irrational pseudoscientific assertions.

Second, you might want to *ask your doctor* about Bendectin because its ingredients can be reproduced over the counter. It's basically made of the antihistamine doxylamine succinate (found in the sleep aid Unisom) and vitamin B6. Bendectin was a time-release medication, so it may be difficult to capture its level of relief, but one could try with peace of mind knowing that the baby will not be harmed. Because the drug is basically an antihistamine, it can make you drowsy, which may be a problem if you have to make a big presentation or be otherwise alert. I guess you have to weigh which is worse: being nauseous or being sleepy. For me, that's a no-brainer, but everyone's different. I am told that the drowsiness is not as bad as taking the motion-sickness drug Dramamine, and it leaves you alert enough to drive a car. I am not advocating that you whip up a batch in your kitchen. I'm just saying you might want to ask your doctor about it.

And, finally, the drug is still available and widely used in Canada, where it's called Diclectin. Because of the numerous studies now saying that Bendectin was unfairly indicted, the Canadian manufacturer Duchesnay is actively working with the FDA to bring the drug back to the U.S. market. We should have it here soon.

Think about it. If you ever find yourself ready to believe morning sickness is an insignificant problem that no one cares about, just remember that the story of one little morning-sickness pill made it all the way to the Supreme

Court and changed the way scientific evidence is admitted into law. As a result, you can rest assured that Bendectin is *the most thoroughly* studied drug there is when it comes to teratogenic effects. In fact, some say Bendectin is the most thoroughly researched and tested drug *ever*.

The loss of Bendectin has left a huge void in our ability to treat morning sickness today in the United States. In an attempt to tally the damage of the loss of this useful drug, both in terms of health and costs, Canadian researchers found that hospital admissions for excessive vomiting in pregnancy rose by as much as 50 percent in 1984 . . . two years after Bendectin was removed from the market. And a rough estimate of related excess hospital costs from 1983 to 1987 was seventy-three million dollars in the United States. The researchers add:

> Such estimates do not take into consideration other costs, such as extra physician vists, increased absenteeism from work, and the effect on quality of life of the pregnant woman and her family. No decrease in rates of congenital malformations could be shown to offset this increased cost to society. (*Canadian Journal of Public Health*, 1995:86/66–70).

Indeed, many doctors in the United States report that they long for a drug like Bendectin and have nothing to offer in its stead. Nothing else has ever really come along to take its place, and chances are that nothing is likely to soon. Persuading drug companies to fund research on drugs for pregnant women is a Herculean task. First of all, there's the thalidomide factor. Second, there's the fear of lawsuits. And third, there's the profit margin to consider. Pregnancy—in particular, morning sickness—is a small market for a big drug company, and pregnant women *are* actually considered an "orphan" population. There are an average of four million live births a year in the United States, and if

Pregnant women are *actually considered an "orphan" population. There are an average of 4 million live births a year in the United States . . . and if only ⅔ to ¾ of pregnant women are suffering morning sickness, it's simply not a big enough population to justify the dollars spent on clinical trials.*

only two-thirds to three-fourths of pregnant women are suffering morning sickness, it's simply not a big enough population to justify the dollars spent on clinical trials.

So for now, we're out of luck in the wonder-drug department. There are a handful of medications used today that have reasonably good safety and efficacy records that you might want to ask your doctor about. Compazine,

Reglan, and Tigan are frequently prescribed. The motion-sickness drug Dramamine has been used extensively in Canada to treat pregnancy-related nausea and vomiting. Some doctors also report success with a drug called Zofran, which is used to control the vomiting caused by chemotherapy. Zofran is what is known as a "Class B" pregnancy drug, meaning that studies in animals indicate that it would also be safe for a pregnant woman to take. There have been some small studies on humans as well, with no reported problems, but more research is warranted for complete confidence in this drug. Zofran is expensive, costing about thirty dollars a pill, and the regime is generally to take it twice a day. I'm not sure if insurance companies would want to pick up the tab for such a pricey morning sickness treatment. Still, feel free to ask your doctor about any of these medications, but be aware that these drugs are known as antiemetics, meaning they only control vomiting . . . and most women with morning sickness will tell you that the nausea is many times worse than the vomiting.

If you are interested in medication, an *excellent* resource is the Canadian organization called "Motherisk." Motherisk specializes in any and all drug-related questions for pregnant women. If you have a question about studies done on a particular drug, it will have the answer. It even has a nausea-and-vomiting hotline you can call and speak to a counselor. Real, live, sympathetic people are standing by on the phones to answer any question you might have relating to morning sickness, from how to handle your feelings to what to eat and what drugs might be safe. The phone number is 1-800-436-8477. Or you can go to their

Motherisk . . . the phone number is 1-800-436-8477. Or you can go to their website: www.motherisk.org.

website: *www.motherisk.org.* I wish I had known about Motherisk when I was pregnant.

Of course . . . no one really wants to take a drug while pregnant, and no one is advocating that you do. I am not a pregnancy pill-pusher. In fact, I had pneumonia during my second pregnancy and was out of my mind with worry about the antibiotics I was forced to swallow so that I could breathe. Every time I popped a couple of Tylenol for a headache, I felt a tinge of guilt and anxiety. But my point is only this: if you're miserable and can't function, there *are* safe things you can try. Let science govern your thinking, not fear. *Ask your doctor.* Have I said that enough?

Dietary Supplements

In the absence of an FDA-approved drug to make our troubles go away, many women with morning sickness are tempted to turn for relief to the world of dietary supplements, herbs, and homeopathic remedies. There's a staggering quantity of information available to both enlighten

If you're miserable and can't function, there are safe things you can try.

and confuse. A search of the Internet turns up dozens of sites from "Moon Dragon Birthing Services" to "Gentlebirth," all of which have long lists of natural herbs to try—and just as many to avoid—during pregnancy. If you are interested in herbal remedies, be certain to stay away from those that are uterine stimulants, abortifacients, or listed as "emmanogogues," which help to regulate menstruation. I found a helpful list of what to avoid on a website called "Snowbound Herbals" (sbherbals.com). Better yet, talk to your doctor.

Dr. Sandy Kweder of the FDA, who specializes in the health of pregnant women, says:

> You have to be careful. There's an assumption that because it's plant-derived or "natural," it is safe. That is not an accurate statement.

Just remember, aspirin is a plant-derived drug; so is digitalis, which can make your heart stop; snake venom is a

> *Be certain to stay away from herbs that are uterine stimu-lants, abortifacients, or listed as "emmanogogues," which help to regulate menstruation.*

natural substance. And the whole world of herbal medi-cines and dietary supplements is not as carefully regulated as pharmaceuticals are. The good news, according to Dr. Kweder, is that there are not many things that have a proven track record of causing major birth defects. If large num-bers of women were taking something extremely dangerous to the fetus, like thalidomide, we would know about it by now. Only you know what degree of risk you want to take.

Having fired off that caveat, the most commonly cited herbs for morning sickness are ginger, chamomile, pepper-mint, raspberry leaf, and wild yam. But hard scientific data on whether or not these substances work, and more impor-tant, whether they are safe, is limited, to say the least. A large-scale analysis of herbal morning-sickness treatments published in the journal *Midwifery* (September, 2000) found that there is *no* consensus in the medical literature to deter-mine that the most commonly taken herbal remedies for morning sickness are safe during pregnancy. The authors searched all major-language medical, nursing, and scien-tific databases, as well as three hundred websites, Internet news groups, books, and magazines. Their conclusion:

Herbal remedies are often seen as safe, drug-free treatments for morning sickness. However, the contradictory information and dearth of original research related to safety indicate that the compounds should be used with caution.

The only two supplements that seem to have the tacit approval of the medical establishment are Vitamin B6 and ginger. B6, also known as pyridoxine, has been prescribed since the 1940s to treat morning sickness, and there is a fair amount of medical literature suggesting that it is safe and effective. As usual, no one is quite sure why or how it works, but the belief is that it helps the body metabolize certain amino acids that may help reduce nausea.

Doctors suggest taking anywhere from twenty-five to fifty milligrams twice a day. Ask your doctor about it. There are lots of good food sources of Vitamin B6, too, if you can choke them down. Try a large banana, brown rice, lean meat and poultry, fish, avocados, whole grains, corn, and nuts. But B6 doesn't work for everybody.

The only two supplements that seem to have the tacit approval of the medical establishment are Vitamin B6 and ginger.

With my first child, I was so nauseated early on that my doctor did an early ultrasound to rule out twins, which I didn't have. But I did try vitamin B6 and B1 shots to help, without much success. The shots only hurt and made my hip sore.   —ELLA D.

There are lots of good food sources of Vitamin B6. Try a large banana, brown rice, lean meat and poultry, fish, avocados, whole grains, corn, and nuts.

Ginger also has a time-worn reputation for relieving the symptoms of morning sickness. The redolent root has been used through the centuries in many Asian cultures as an aid to digestion and a stomach soother, and ginger ale remains one of the old standbys for relieving nausea and stomach upset. But much of what we know about ginger is still folklore. One of the few scientific studies of ginger's effectiveness was recently published in the journal *Obstetrics and Gynecology* (April 2001). The study looked at seventy women. Thirty-two of them were given 250 milligrams of powdered ginger three times a day after meals and one before bedtime, and thirty-eight were given a placebo. After four days, 90 percent of the women who took the ginger reported a decrease in the severity of nausea, versus 29 percent who took the placebo. That is *not* to say that the nausea went away, but that the symptoms were lessened without side effects or risks to the fetus.

My objection to ginger is that it is strong-smelling and stronger-tasting. In the early days of my pregnancies, my mother showed up proffering large bottles of ginger capsules, and just the thought of trying to swallow one was too much to bear. I couldn't stomach it. However, I did have strong cravings for and found great relief from several Chinese dishes, many of which are prepared with ginger. Perhaps eating ginger cooked into foods is the best way to get it into your system. But if you can handle straight ginger and your doctor thinks it's a safe choice, try it; it comes up often on the list of potential remedies. Be aware, though, that megadoses of *anything* can be harmful. That's why all the studies involve small quantities. It's a safe way to start.

If you don't want to subject the developing fetus to any kind of drug or herb, acupuncture is an option. But doctors caution that acupuncture, if performed improperly, can induce premature labor. There are certain acupuncture points that can stimulate uterine contractions. If you are considering acupuncture, be sure to discuss it with your doctor first. Acupuncture has certainly gained a degree of acceptance in the medical community over the years. It has even been endorsed by the National Institutes of Health as an alternative or complement to some standard medical treatments. But does it work for relieving morning sickness? Results of the most recent studies are curiously contradictory. Some researchers say that acupuncture is no more effec-

Be aware that megadoses of **anything** *can be harmful.*

tive than being poked by a cocktail stick. Literally. A study, published in April of 2001 by the American College of Obstetricians and Gynecologists (ACOG), compared the use of acupuncture on pregnant women suffering nausea versus what's known in the medical-study world as a "sham" treatment; in this case, the women were pricked with cocktail sticks. Fifty-five women were in the study, not a huge number, but the conclusion was that those given genuine acupuncture had no more relief from their nausea than those treated with cocktail sticks. A much bigger and more recent study, done at the University of Adelaide in Australia, found just the opposite. In that study, said to be the world's first comprehensive study of the use of acupuncture to treat morning sickness, six hundred women were tested. The women, all less than fourteen weeks pregnant, were each given weekly twenty-minute sessions of acupuncture for four weeks. The treatment involved a combination of acupuncture points on the forearm, lower leg, below the knee, the foot, and the abdomen. The results, published in the American journal *Birth* in March of 2002, found that the relief from nausea was significant and that women who received even one acupuncture session felt better.

The things we do to try to understand this ailment.

If you don't want to be poked with needles, or cocktail

sticks, for that matter, something else to try that is noninvasive and drug-free is acupressure bands that you wear on your wrist. Some are called "reliefbands"; others, to control motion sickness, are called "seabands." You have nothing to lose from trying them because they are safe. But to be perfectly honest, in my anecdotal gathering of information of women who tried them, I have never ever heard one say *"Eureka! Seabands! I'm cured!"* I do believe they can soften symptoms with the power of suggestion, but can they overpower a full-blown case of morning sickness? You be the judge.

One other unusual treatment found on the Internet is something called the "Morning Well for Morning Sickness"—a registered medical device. As described in promotional literature, it is "a simple audio-cassette tape containing a revolutionary audio programme that has been created from a unique blend of music, specific frequencies and pulses to cure the symptoms of morning sickness." I guess this device is based on the theory that morning sickness is caused by imbalances in the vestibular system—the part of your inner ear that controls balance—and soothing the ear with music and pulses could bring it all back to normal. I'm skeptical. But then, I'm a natural skeptic because I'm a reporter. The device is drug-free, noninvasive, and I guess has just as much potential as any other New Age panacea. Try it!

Rest and Avoidance

Before you spend money on a new device to normalize your vestibular dysfunction, bear in mind that some of the best ways to treat morning sickness are often the simplest. Get LOTS of rest. Many women report that the only time they are ever free of the nausea is when they are asleep, so nap, rest, sleep as much as your life will allow. Easier said than done, I know. But make sleep a priority.

Another big help is *avoidance*! In other words, try to track the triggers that bring on your worse cases of nausea and vomiting and *avoid* them. If it's the smell of meat cooking, for heaven's sake, don't allow meat to be cooked in your house. Go out for dinner if your kids are clamoring for hamburgers or your husband wants a steak. Or let them go out by themselves; the peace and quiet might be good for you. If it's perfume and deodorant? Don't wear it. My absolute favorite scent made me gag when I was pregnant, so I gave it up. Get the carpets and curtains cleaned. Avoid hot, stuffy, enclosed spaces. Leave your windows open. Stress is also a major trigger for bad bouts of nausea. Whenever possible, try to make this early part of your pregnancy as stress-free as

The best ways to treat morning sickness are often the simplest. Get LOTS of rest.

possible. If you're a type-A overachiever, step back and relax for a while. If you're a harried, working mother, try to accept the reality that you may not be on the top of your professional game for a few months and that your house might not be as clean as usual. Ask for help. Delegate. Admit that you feel lousy and need a rest. Avoiding stress is good for your health and the health of your growing baby.

Track the triggers that bring on your worse cases of nausea and vomiting and avoid them.

Of course, some things are difficult to avoid, like life. You can't just sequester yourself in a sweet-smelling, white-padded cell and lie down all day. But to the best of your ability, chip away at anything you don't need to do that might make you feel that little bit better. Remember, it's all about survival.

Avoid hot, stuffy, enclosed spaces. Leave your windows open.

8

Food: Don't Leave Home Without It

The only time I threw up was the first morning I tried saltine crackers. —MARY PAT L.

In thinking about the structure of this book, I really wanted to include food in the chapter on treatment because, in my opinion, the only thing that really ever works in keeping the dreadful symptoms of morning sickness at bay is *eating.* The best advice I think I could ever give anyone who has morning sickness, and certainly the best advice ever given to me, is: always have food nearby, eat many small meals or snacks all day long, and *never* let your stomach be empty. Is there scientific evidence proving that this strategy is the answer? Nope. Is there anecdotal evidence? Lots. Certainly enough to warrant storing granola bars and pretzels in your purse the way a squirrel stores nuts for the winter. Being able to eat in that split second when you start feeling shaky or sweaty or nauseous can mean the difference between throwing up in public or escaping, albeit narrowly, with your dignity intact.

Part of the struggle with food, though, is that if you're nauseous, you don't always want to eat, so picking the right

The best advice I think I could ever give anyone who has morning sickness, and certainly the best advice ever given to me, is: always have food nearby, eat many small meals or snacks all day long, and never let your stomach be empty. Being able to eat in that split second when you start feeling shaky or sweaty or nauseous can mean the difference between throwing up in public or escaping, albeit narrowly, with your dignity intact.

food at the right time is yet another challenge. For some unknown reason, during morning sickness nothing ever tastes quite right, and foods you once loved all of a sudden turn on you. This can lead to one of the more bizarre and disturbing side effects of morning sickness, something I came to call "food indecision." I pride myself on being able to make quick and sound decisions in my normal life, and yet for some reason, during the four months of my morning sickness, the question, Turkey or ham-and-cheese?, became as significant an existential dilemma as "to be or not to be."

And then when I finally decided what I wanted, I had to have it that very second. I would walk around the CBS cafeteria in circles for a half an hour just trying to decide what looked good, what I could stomach on that particular day. It was often the same thing over and over again, but I had to consider everything first because I was so afraid of eating the wrong thing. It's also disturbing because while food is clearly one of life's great pleasures, no one wants to be held hostage to it. While you're in that morning meeting, you'd like to be able to concentrate on the business at hand instead of counting the minutes until you can tear into that package of graham crackers stashed (wisely, I might add) in your desk drawer. But morning sickness changes all that.

I would describe my relationship with food during my morning sickness as being food-obsessed. I seemed to be always planning my next meal or snack, hopeful that I would eat something that would make me feel less nauseated.   —CHRISTINE H.

Obsessions with food exacerbate the feeling of being out of control that seizes so many women with morning sickness. We will go to great lengths to get that one food that will make us feel better. I once left two huge piles of laundry sitting on our bed one Saturday afternoon and disappeared without a trace to go in search of hot-and-sour soup, which on any other day of the week would have made me ill. Our home looked like the scene of an abduction: door left open, TV on, laundry strewn all over, and me happily down the street at Shun-Lee West slurping up a big bowl of hot-and-sour soup all by myself.

One night on my way home from work, I got the most extreme craving for canned corn. I had no cash and the supermarket had a ten-dollar minimum for debit cards. So I ended up buying a shopping cart full of useless food items to allow me to purchase my seventy-nine-cent can of corn. It was so satisfying, though.
—PAXTON B.

. . . I did make my husband take me out to a diner at ten o'clock at night so I could have mashed potatoes and gravy. —SUSAN S.

One night I awoke during my third pregnancy craving spaghetti sauce with meatballs and too tired to heat it up. I stood in the dark and drank a small jar straight from the refrigerator. I felt like the woman in Rosemary's Baby . . . I needed tomatoes constantly that entire pregnancy. —CHRISTINE K.

And that brings me to what may be the most important point I can stress about food. When you are suffering from morning sickness, *you should eat whatever works!* It may be steaks and baked potatoes. It may be butterscotch candy and rootbeer, it may be cold spaghetti sauce in the middle of the night, but the bottom line is that you need to keep something in your stomach that will help you survive. In most cases, the baby will be fine. Remember, early on, your developing child is an embryo no bigger than the size of a pea. It doesn't need much food, but *you* need to stay hydrated and able to summon the strength to carry this baby to term. In her book *Eating For Two: The Complete Guide to Nutrition During Pregnancy*, Nancy Abbott Hess, a dietician, writes:

> Eat whatever you can, even if that means nothing but ginger ale, Popsicles, and hard candy . . . your digestive system is very resourceful at capturing calories.

This is a crucial point because women, *especially* pregnant women, seem to have a genetic tendency to be consumed by guilt about whatever they consume. Will I put on too much weight? Will the baby get all the vitamins he or she needs? Am I eating too much fat? Too little calcium?

One of the best-selling books on pregnancy, *What to Expect When You're Expecting,"* advocates something

When you are suffering from morning sickness, you should eat WHATEVER works!

called the "best odds diet," rich in foods like kale and sweet potatoes and broccoli. I found this diet incredibly frustrating. It's all well and good if you don't have morning sickness. But just the thought of eating kale and broccoli turned me the equivalent shade of green, and as a result, I often felt guilty and inadequate. What was wrong with me that I couldn't eat vegetables? Why were the only things I could choke down—cheeseburgers, peanut butter, and bread—all high in fat and carbohydrates? It's hard giving in to your cravings under the watchful eye of the fat-free, low-cholesterol world in which we live, but for this fleeting period in your life, you really have to give up on those basic food groups and feel free to turn the food pyramid upside down and eat what works for you.

As a nonpregnant woman, I am extremely conscious of what I eat. I avoid artificial ingredients, food dyes, fatty foods, fast foods, and try to eat pesticide/hormone-free food. I am slender and healthy. During this bout with morning sickness, I have craved salty, greasy fast food: Filet-O-Fish from McDonald's, french fries,

ketchup, french onion soup with lots of crusty moz-
zarella melted on top, turkey sandwiches with lots of
mayo, feta cheese, garlic shrimp, to name a few. These
cravings were nearly frenzied for me, and fulfilling one
was like breathing after holding my breath. —LU H.

Remember: *guilt is a dirty word*! You can always return
to your healthy, normal diet once you get through this
period, and chances are that you will do it without missing
a beat. But what is the point in fighting heart disease after
all if your pregnancy kills you first? Try to look at the bright
side of whatever your guilty pleasure is. Instead of thinking
cheese equals fat, think cheese equals calcium. Instead of
thinking cheeseburger equals heart attack, think cheeseburger equals protein. French fries *are* vegetables! Are
there low-fat, low-cholesterol sources of calcium and protein? Of course, and if you want them, go ahead. If not,
though, ingest and enjoy!

I enjoyed chocolate eclairs and poached salmon.
                                                    —RUTH K.

Stouffer's Turkey Tetrazzini—that was the best
advice I got. My best friend recommended it. It has
meat (so to speak), and it is warm and comforting.
This food literally saved me. —PAXTON B.

Instead of thinking cheese equals fat, think cheese equals cal-
cium. Instead of thinking cheeseburger equals heart attack,
think cheeseburger equals protein. French fries are vegetables!

I had this craving for cheese Whoppers at Burger King.
Those I could eat, and the greasy french fries and the
sweet Coke. The heavy combination coated and filled
my stomach and yet didn't make me throw up and feel
nauseous. I don't know why. For the first five months of
the pregnancies, I went to Burger King almost every
single day for lunch . . . I didn't worry about it.

—MARY JANE C.

Having advised you to eat what you like and crave, I
acknowledge that finding that perfect food can be difficult
and you have to be a little inventive. That odd metallic taste
in your mouth seems to taint every other flavor, so it can be
hard to eat with gusto. In fact, many women complain they
can't even drink water when they have morning sickness.

Food was a constant battle and source of simultaneous
obsession and disappointment. I would get the idea

*that pizza would satisfy my hunger and relieve nau-
sea, only to find that it did neither. Carbs seemed allur-
ing: potatoes, bread, chips, pasta, oatmeal . . . I
would eat these items in rotation and feel overly full
and unsatisfied afterward.*   —CHRIS S.

*Celery, french fries, and ice cream were some of the
things that were okay to eat. I later found out that my
grandmother ate celery to fight morning sickness.*
          —KERRY M.

To find the right foods, morning sickness expert and
registered dietician Miriam Erick suggests that you think
about foods in terms of their characteristics. In other
words, instead of asking yourself, Will this banana make
me feel better? ask, Do I want a food that is sweet and yel-
low? Or one that is orange and tart? Would I rather have
something salty and crunchy? When food just doesn't taste
the way it should, you might find it helpful to "boil" things
down to their most basic elements.

The following categories seem to cover most foods:

SALTY	SPICY
CRUNCHY	LIQUID
FRUITY	HOT
SOUR	TART
SMOOTH	SOLID

BLAND	COLD
BITTER	TANGY
WET	LUMPY
EARTHY	TEMPERATE
SWEET	FIZZY
DRY	CREAMY

That old cliché about pregnant women wanting pickles and ice cream together has many variations; it's all about wanting a combination of textures and tastes: salty and crunchy, and sweet and creamy! Erick also suggests keeping a food diary so you can remember which combinations of flavors and textures worked for you at particular times of day, and you can also keep track of which foods make you nauseous.

And just a little pointer, something I am sure you've already discovered if you've been vomiting at all: try to choose foods that won't be completely horrible coming back up. I know it's disgusting, but we have to get things out in the open here in the name of self-preservation. Stay away from grape juice, long pasta noodles, beets, and fudge brownies. You get the picture. Enough said.

It didn't matter what I ate, I always threw up or felt awful. Mandarin oranges, applesauce, toast, poached eggs, Jell-O, pears—all aren't too bad coming back up!
—LORI S.

Keep a food diary so you can remember which combinations of flavors and textures worked for you at particular times of day, and you can also keep track of which foods make you nauseous.

As discussed in the chapter looking at evolutionary theories for why morning sickness exists, surveys suggest that there are categories of foods that inspire passionate aversions . . . and similar categories of foods that women crave. In my gathering of information, I have found that one food group that consistently seems to help is fruit and fruit juice.

A typical workday: I got up and ate six oranges, each like it was my last.   —ELIZABETH P. G.

My favorite foods were grapefruit and watermelon . . . and later, jelly beans!   —PAM E.

Perhaps, as our evolutionary theorists suggest, it's because fruit contains fewer microorganisms and phytochemicals than their leafy green cousins. Perhaps it's just because fruit is cold and sweet, crispy and tart, and good for you! Whatever the reason, I couldn't get enough icy-cold watermelon and pineapple through the summer, and crunchy apples in the fall. I found orange juice too acidic but craved lemonade. One fallback I could always count on to get me through the morning was a big bowl of fruit salad and cottage cheese. If fresh fruit seems like too much washing, peeling, or chewing, you can even try canned fruit. I found canned fruit cocktail and canned pears mixed with yogurt particularly soothing, and if you buy the kind in natural juice, or if you rinse off the sugary syrup, it's a reasonably healthy snack. So, if I may make one suggestion about what to try, it is fruit. It helped me through some tough spots, and mercifully, it is one food group that's healthy, so you don't have to feel guilt about indulging in it.

And now a few words from the experts. I thought I would share some of the unusual food cravings, food thoughts, and food "treatments," if you will, that other women shared with me. Try them . . . or run screaming!

Everywhere I went, I carried saltines, a bottle of water, and antacids. I also started off my days with protein: yogurt, oatmeal, eggs. This helped the most.
                                        —JENNIFER W.

Eggs and cheese, especially in combination, seemed to make me have better days.   —AMY C.

I had not been a meat eater. I did not have a real meal with red meat for about fifteen years. That all changed when I got pregnant. I craved meat and I ate it. From that point on, I have been a full-fledged meat eater.
                                                    —HILARY T.

Bologna sandwiches with enough mayonnaise to sink a battleship . . . and gas-station Hostess SnoBalls . . . pink icing with coconut covering chocolate cupcakes.
                                                    —JENNY E.

Venison salami   —MELISSA T.

Bean burritos from Taco Bell. (I never eat at fast-food places.)   —ANONYMOUS

Peanut butter and banana sandwiches, peanut butter and salami sandwiches, rocky-road ice cream with orange pop.   —RAQUEL T.

Those candy orange slices (jelly candy coated in sugar) . . . for some reason, I really loved them and would eat a whole bag. Also I loved cantaloupe. I could eat a whole one.   —LORI S.

One thing I really enjoyed was root beer: root beer Popsicles, root-beer floats. Yum!   —DONNA B.

I craved potato pierogies with cottage cheese. I had never eaten this combination before but found that I

was making this meal (for myself only) at least three times a week throughout the pregnancy.   —LAURA P.

I craved very unhealthy foods: macaroni and cheese, grilled cheese sandwiches, pasta. I ate a lot of soup and I carried almonds, eating a few almonds every few minutes to always maintain a bit of protein in my stomach. That helped.   —ANONYMOUS

One morning I ate chopped chicken livers with a french-fry chaser.   —MICHELLE

I ate gallons and gallons of mocha-chip ice cream. I ate a ton of peanut butter. I would have a grilled cheese sandwich for lunch and then go have another.
     —ANN C.

I ate whitefish and a bagel almost every morning. Next, I had a hankering for turkey on English muffins.
     —JODIE G.

I was a lifelong Coca-Cola "addict," and I could not look at a Coke. I literally had to turn off Coke ads. I started drinking Perrier with lime or 7UP.   —LAURA P.

I ate bag after bag of pretzel nuggets and drank tons of cherry Gatorade. I was very, very thirsty and for the first time in my life, I was repulsed by water.
     —CARYN R.

I craved junk food as if I had a bad hangover. McDonald's made me feel better at 11:00 A.M. I had to have a Coke (not diet) every day . . . also, frozen grapes and bananas really helped nausea.

—LOUISA W.

The only clear memory I have is needing to eat before I picked up my head off the pillow each morning.

—CATHY C.

Just carbos . . . but after the fourth month, my husband called me "hoss" 'cause I ate entire club sandwiches, hoagies, and a serving of anything from Denny's.

—MARY G.

I don't like apples, yet I craved them. I haven't had an apple since I gave birth. I wanted Sugar Smacks cereal so badly one night I screamed at my husband. He went to the store with a friend, and my husband and friend each bought me a box of Sugar Smacks.   —PAT L.

Pitted prunes filled with peanut butter.   —PEGGY L.

I would sip warm Jell-O . . . any color.

—KRISTEN C.

I felt like I couldn't go a day in my second and third trimesters without Oreo cookies. I'm sure that's why my daughter loves them today.   —SUSAN S.

Rice cakes with cheese, melted in the microwave at work. My coworkers got suspicious about my pregnancy when I started eating this snack twice a day.

—JENNY L.

Besides chocolate-chip ice cream with pickles, I would squeeze lemon juice on tortilla chips.

—ELIZABETH G.

While working during my second pregnancy, I would sneak out of the office at around 10:00 A.M., and walk to the new building site down the street where a vendor canteen truck would serve the construction crew. I would order a ham-and-cheese or bologna sandwich (sometimes two) and eat them on the spot. While at home during my third pregnancy, I would have a chicken alfredo frozen entree every morning, also around 10:00 A.M.   —CHRISTINE H.

I almost drank the pickle juice from a jar I had just polished off, but stopped myself, realizing that this was just a bit much.   —HEATHER S.

All I can add to this remarkable menu is: You never know until you try it.

9

Exercise to Exorcise

Working out was one of the few things that ever made me feel like my old self again . . . even if just for an hour.   —BETSEY D.

I can say with some certainty that the period during which you are suffering morning sickness will be like no other in your life. Nothing tastes the same, smells the same, looks the same, or feels the same. It's a bizarre episode of sensory upheaval in which foods you once loved seem abhorrent and things you would never normally eat, you crave with gusto. Yet there is one thing that, at least for me, was a constant between my non-nauseous world and my nauseous world, and that was exercise. I am not and never have been a gym fanatic. I like to exercise, but I do it because I have to, and for the most part, I am one of those people who needs to stay disciplined and focused about going to the gym or it's not going to happen. Let's just say I love my workout . . . when it's all over. But I have to say, too, that exercising during morning sickness was a sanctuary for me. My prenatal exercise class on Saturday mornings was the only thing that consistently offered me an hour of relief from my all-consuming nausea. It became something I actually looked forward to rather than dreaded, as I did most other activities in my months of misery.

I am imagining a roar of groans from readers, and I realize the call to exercise may be hard to hear because, of course, it requires that rarest of commodities during morning sickness—energy. But it does help! If it made you feel better *before* you were pregnant, guess what: exercise will make you feel better *during* your pregnancy. Of course, before you even stretch your arms over your head and take a deep breath, you must *ask your doctor* about an exercise program. This is especially important for women having

The American College of Obstetricians and Gynecologists (ACOG) issued new exercise guidelines in January of 2002 suggesting that pregnant women "engage in 30 minutes or more of moderate exercise on most, if not all, days of the week."

high-risk pregnancies. But in general, exercise during pregnancy is considerred perfectly safe and is, in fact, recommended. The American College of Obstetricians and Gynecologists (ACOG) issued new exercise guidelines in January of 2002 suggesting that pregnant women "engage in 30 minutes or more of moderate exercise on most, if not all, days of the week." Just be reasonable about it and stay in tune with your body. Don't start vigorous workouts because you think it might make your morning sickness disappear. And just in case you were tempted, ACOG also suggests that you avoid the following sports while pregnant: kick boxing, ice hockey, soccer, horseback riding, and scuba diving! As we like to joke in the medical journalism business, "This, from the Medical Journal. *Duh.*"

Once you have started, there are some warning signs to keep in the front of your mind. If you experience any of the following, you should stop exercising and contact your doctor:

- VAGINAL BLEEDING
- DYSPNEA PRIOR TO EXERTION
- DIZZINESS
- HEADACHE
- CHEST PAIN
- MUSCLE WEAKNESS
- CALF PAIN OR SWELLING
- PRE-TERM LABOR
- DECREASED FETAL MOVEMENT
- AMNIOTIC FLUID LEAKAGE

Once you have started, you might notice that you feel better right away. Part of the relief is, of course, no mystery. Those famous exercise hormones called "endorphins" kick in, leading to what some have termed an exercise "high." Endorphins are just as active during pregnancy as before, and they can fight their way through the fog of morning sickness and make you feel good about yourself in general. Endorphins have a chemical structure similar to the pain-killing drug morphine. Morphine acts

If you experience any of the following, you should stop exercising and contact your doctor:

- *vaginal bleeding*
- *dyspnea prior to exertion*
- *dizziness*
- *headache*
- *chest pain*
- *muscle weakness*
- *calf pain or swelling*
- *pre-term labor*
- *decreased fetal movement*
- *amniotic fluid leakage*

on specific sites in the brain and spinal cord called "opiate receptors," dulling them and, in turn, the sensation of pain. Endorphins also act on the body's opiate receptors. In fact, the word "endorphin" is short for "endogenous morphine," endogenous meaning something the body produces on its own.

There are many other physical benefits. Have you ever noticed that when you feel nauseous or queasy, it sometimes helps to take big, deep breaths, get out in the fresh air, or maybe even put your head down between your knees to breathe in? That's because oxygen helps! Getting as much oxygen as possible can make the head-spinning, dizziness, and sweatiness subside, at least temporarily. Exercise increases the flow of oxygen into your lungs, into your bloodstream, and into your brain, and that has the capacity to soften the symptoms of morning sickness. Also, getting more oxygen and pumping up your heart rate a little bit could help you feel less sluggish. There is a natural inclination when you are feeling lousy to want to lie around and do nothing, and who can blame you? But that tends to create a negative feedback loop: you feel lousy so you don't do anything, and then you feel worse because you're not doing anything. Getting up and moving might help a little with the inertia.

But it's not just about oxygen. From the moment you conceive, your body begins to undergo a series of physical changes to prepare you for the hard work of carrying a baby for nine months and then delivering that baby. First, a hormone called "relaxin" kicks in to loosen up your ligaments. Relaxin is critical for allowing the body to survive the trauma of childbirth, but in the process, it also makes pregnant women a little wobbly. You may discover that all of your major joints, like your ankles, wrists, and knees, get loose and you are not so stable on your feet. According to pregnancy-fitness expert Peggy Levine, who runs the pre-natal exercise studio in New York City that saved my life, as your belly begins to grow, your pelvis will start to tilt for-ward to accommodate the shift in weight and as a result, the ligaments known as the "hip flexors" start to get shorter. As the gravity of a growing baby pulls you down, you may experience lower back pain, your arches may drop, your shoulders may ache, your alignment will be redesigned, and your whole sense of equilibrium may be off. Any good, carefully taught prenatal exercise class will focus both on stretching and aerobic activity, because while the stretching can help ease your body through all physical changes, the aerobic activity will get that needed oxygen into your system.

A lot of people swear by pregnancy yoga classes, which focus exclusively on stretching the body and calming the mind. These classes have become increasingly popular and as a result, increasingly available. If you've been advised not to do a lot of cardiovascular exercise during your preg-nancy, yoga would be an excellent choice for you and could really help with the "mind-over-matter" element of surviv-ing morning sickness. In addition, A lot of women suffer heartburn and something called acid reflux along with their morning sickness. Peggy Levine says that stretching the abdomen, keeping the body as elongated as possible, can help ease the effects of the reflux.

On the whole, staying stretched out and limber may not directly address the problem of morning sickness and nausea, but pregnancy comes hand in hand with many physical discomforts, and they can often become indistinguishable. Let's call it general pregnancy malaise. If your body is achy and creaky and wobbly and out of alignment *and* you feel nauseous, solving one problem may help with the others. It has been my experience that deep stretching and deep breathing contribute to an overall feeling of well-being that takes away some of the discomfort of morning sickness. At least temporarily.

In many ways, exercise during morning sickness is better medicine for the head than for the body. Much of my struggle with morning sickness revolved around the fact that I felt completely out of control. I didn't trust my body anymore, couldn't eat the things I normally liked, and could barely function. Exercise was one thing that restored a modicum of control to my life. It gave me some sense of being in charge of my body rather than my body running the show. It also got me "out of myself." With music blaring and other pregnant women by my side bopping to the beat, I was freed from dwelling on every unpleasant physical sensation and could just have fun. People exercise to stay fit, but just as many do it to escape their troubles and stress. The same applies during morning sickness. At least for me, for one hour my body did as it was told, I wasn't obsessed with my misery, and I left Peggy Levine Studio feeling like I might be able to make it through another day.

A few words of advice: even though they are all made of Lycra and spandex and can probably stretch, don't try to cram yourself into your pre-pregnancy workout gear. All that elastic cutting into your belly and anywhere else you are growing will only make you feel uncomfortable and

> *Be sure to eat something solid and filling before your work-*
> *out. A bagel and cream cheese, or whole-wheat toast and*
> *peanut butter, will do the trick. And be sure to drink plenty*
> *of fluids before and after.*

self-conscious, and it will limit your mobility. There are beautiful maternity exercise clothes on the market, or better yet, try a baggy old pair of sweatpants and a T-shirt. Also, be sure to eat something solid and filling before your workout. A bagel and cream cheese, or whole-wheat toast and peanut butter, will do the trick. And be sure to drink plenty of fluids before and after.

I have nothing but empathy and understanding for those of you who can't get off the couch, but I offer exercise as something to try as a potential break from your trials and tribulations. Every little bit helps. You can even go for a nice brisk walk around the block: just fill your lungs with fresh air and your mind with thoughts of that beautiful baby nestled safely inside you.

FIGURE 1: DEEP BREATHING STRETCH

- OPENS AND EXPANDS LUNGS
- STRETCHES AND LOOSENS LOWER BACK
- ENGAGES AND STRENGTHENS ABDOMINAL MUSCLES

1. Start in a hips' width parallel standing position and inhale with arms stretched out to sides approximately shoulder height.

2. Slowly exhale and pull your arms in front of you as though you were hugging a beach ball, using your abdominals to pull your pelvis under your shoulders.

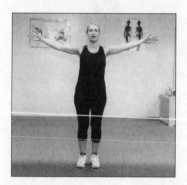 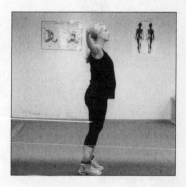

3. Drop your head, drop your shoulders, and round your upper back forward.

4. Inhale and reverse this stretch until your arms are back out by your sides, your back is upright, and head and shoulders are lifted.

5. Repeat several times until your back feels loose and you have taken several good, deep breaths.

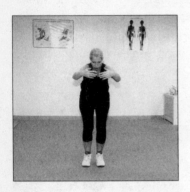 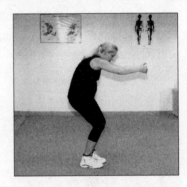

FIGURE 2: SQUAT SPIRALS

- OPENS UP CHEST
- STRETCHES AND STRENGTHENS INNER THIGHS AND HAMSTRINGS
- OPENS AND EXPANDS LUNGS
- LOOSENS LIGAMENTS AND HIP FLEXORS

1. In a squatting position, with the upper body angled forward, place hands on thighs or knees. First inhale, then gently twist upper body to the right while exhaling and engaging abdominals. Hold for several seconds.

2. Inhale as you gently twist your body back through the center and exhale, and engage abdominals again as your upper body spirals to the left.

3. Repeat several times.

4. Return upper body to center and slowly stand, rolling the body up one vertebra at a time during an exhalation.

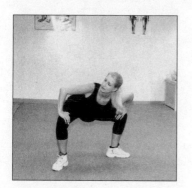 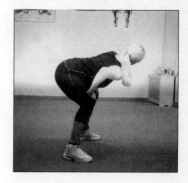

FIGURE 3: LATERAL STRETCH

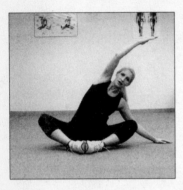

- EXPANDS AND OPENS LUNGS
- STRETCHES SPINE AND SIDES
- LOOSENS HIPS
- GIVES YOUR BABY AND YOUR ORGANS MORE ROOM
- RELEASES NECK AND SHOULDER TENSION

1. Start sitting with soles of feet together.

2. Keep chest lifted and shoulders dropped. Inhale.

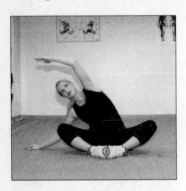 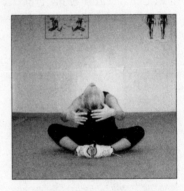

3. Reaching one arm out to your side on the floor, stretch the other up over the head, and as you exhale bend gently to the side so that the elbow of the outstretched arm reaches toward the floor, touching if you can and if it's comfortable.

4. Hold the stretch while inhaling and exhaling. Always use your "abdominal hug" to return upright.

5. Repeat stretch to other side.

FIGURE 4: "CAT AND COW" STRETCH

- STRETCHES BACK
- USES AND TIGHTENS ABDOMINALS
- RELEASES HIP, NECK, AND SHOULDER TENSION

1. Start on hands and knees. Inhale.

2. On an exhale, gently round back upward and your head and neck down, like a cat stretching, and hold.

3. On the inhale, relax the stretch and bring your tailbone (also known as "sitz bone") up toward the ceiling so that your lower back is eased in the opposite direction and hold your head up, looking forward, careful not to overstretch abdominals.

4. Repeat several times.

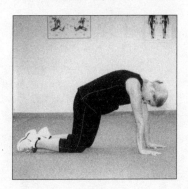 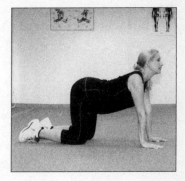

FIGURE 5: RESTING STRETCH, ALSO KNOWN AS "CHILD'S POSE" IN YOGA

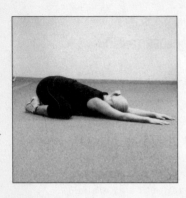

- STRETCHES ARMS AND SIDES
- STRETCHES QUADRUCEPS, HAMSTRINGS, AND BUTTOCKS
- BRINGS BREATHING AND HEART RATE BACK TO NORMAL
- RELAXES BODY AND *MIND*

1. From the previous cat back stretch, simply spread your knees out to the sides, reach arms forward, and lay body down as far as your belly and muscles will allow. Keep head down and continue inhaling and exhaling.

2. Hold as long as you want. (You may never get up!)

10

A Short Word About Prenatal Vitamins

My food secret was taking the vitamins with plain old-fashioned oatmeal. It really worked. —JENNIFER W.

YUCK!

Well, that's not really the short word I was thinking of, but it does kind of sum it up. Can you imagine anything worse than feeling chronically nauseous, having a tough time finding anything to eat that doesn't make you gag, and being told to swallow a giant medicine-y-smelling-and-tasting horse pill? What are they thinking? Is this all part of that great male conspiracy out there scheming to make women suffer?

On top of everything else I was going through, I felt a nagging sense of guilt and failure that I could *not, no way, no how,* take that prenatal vitamin that was going to make my child superior in every way. I tried and tried and tried, but couldn't face it. There were days when I would stand at the sink with the pill in my fingers, lift my fingers to my lips, shudder . . . and slam-dunk the thing down the drain.

But if you're like me, don't fret. There are a few solutions.

First, never *ever* try to take vitamins on an empty stomach. I know some people say they lose their effectiveness if taken with food or with milk, but forget about all that for now. Shove one in a cube of cheddar cheese, the way you would give a pill to your cat. Take them with whatever works, but *not* on an empty stomach.

Second, try taking your vitamins at night, or at any time

First, never ever *try to take vitamins on an empty stomach.*

of day when you have a lull in the action, so to speak. If lunchtime is an hour of relative stability for you and you've got that big old comforting grilled-cheese sandwich in your stomach, make sure the vitamins are handy so you can pop one in whenever you have the intestinal fortitude to do so. Also, cut your pills in half if you can and take them in pieces.

If you really can't manage the prescription version, my

Try taking your vitamins at night.

obstetrician suggested I try Flintstone's vitamins, or the equivalent. For one thing, you can suck on them and they're not offensive-tasting: sort of like a SweeTARTS. For another, since they're made for children, they are not hard on the stomach. I realize that they are not designed for pregnant women and you may feel like they are not fulfilling your or your baby's needs, but they *do* supply you with 50 percent of the RDA (Recommended Daily Allowance) of vitamins and minerals for an *adult*. Keep reminding yourself that something is better than nothing.

Another great substitute is Total cereal. Cereal was a big morning-sickness food for me. Something about the icy-cold milk and the crunchy flakes was appealing, so eating Total was easy. It has 100 percent of the RDA of major vitamins and minerals.

While all vitamins and minerals are important, the most crucial reason for taking those nasty prenatals is folic acid:

Try Flintstone's vitamins.

a compound of the vitamin B groups and naturally found in leafy green vegetables, oranges, beans, liver, and yeast. There is compelling evidence that folic acid can prevent birth defects known as neural-tube defects, in which the spinal cord and brain of the embryo don't develop normally. Spina bifida, in which the backbones do not form a protective ring around the spinal cord, is one of the most common neural-tube defects, but there are a variety of other problems that can occur. Folic acid appears to have such a profound ability to reduce the risk of these birth defects that the government now requires food manufacturers to put it in our food. It's found in breads and cereals, and even in potato chips. At last—a good reason to eat potato chips. The Centers for Disease Control reported in June of 2001 that since the folic-acid fortification program has been in place, neural-tube defects have declined 20 percent, meaning that eight hundred fewer babies with

The Centers for Disease Control reported in June of 2001 that since the folic-acid fortification program has been in place, neural-tube defects have declined 20 percent, meaning that 800 fewer babies with birth defects are born every year as a result. So even if you absolutely can't take a multivitamin in any form, TAKE FOLIC ACID!

birth defects are born every year as a result. So even if you absolutely can't take a multivitamin in any form, *Take folic acid!* You can buy capsules of it at the health food store and open them up and sprinkle the contents onto whatever food you can eat: applesauce, yogurt, even ice cream.

And if you are reading this book in anticipation of becoming pregnant, start taking folic acid *now*. I always felt anxious that I couldn't take the vitamins when I was pregnant, but there was comfort in knowing that I took them for the six months before I woke up with that queasy feeling.

11

In Sickness and in Health

*It was frustrating. I think my husband thought I was
crazy . . .* —CLAUDIA O'C.

If there is one person as immobi-
lized by morning sickness as the woman who is going
through it, it is her husband or partner. All of a sudden, his
vibrant companion, the person he dreamed of having children with, is a shadow of her former self, most often
screaming "Don't touch me!" or "I want Kung Pao
chicken . . . *now!*" Where she was once neatly dressed and
groomed, she is neglecting to brush her hair and teeth, and
if she was upbeat and confident, she no longer feels like
leaving the house. It's hard on any relationship, and especially hard on the most intimate of partnerships because
while the husband is experiencing it, he's not *really* feeling

it. It is hard to articulate what it's like to be nauseous all the time, but most men *have* had some experience with stomach flu, food poisoning, or too much tequila and can dredge up those memories for a little empathy.

Sex, of course, can become a particularly contentious issue. It can be hard to feel all slinky and amorous when you're worried about keeping your dinner down. On the other hand, some women report being extra interested, with all those good pregnancy juices flowing. I know it's the oldest advice in the book, but do talk about it so that you both have the same expectations.

Sex was not very comfortable during the early months, and that was when he couldn't understand my unreadiness.   —CHRISTINE K.

My husband did the dishes, laundry, and handled the cooking/grilling/sautéing of meat (which could make me hurl in a New York minute). He's been wonderful.
    —LU H.

The house my husband and I were living in at the time had one bathroom that was being renovated. There was clutter, dust, building materials all over the upstairs where the bathroom was located. My husband played hockey in a men's league and it was clear to me that he just wanted to get out of the house while I really wanted him to stay and hold me because I felt so sick. I was sit-

ting on the dirty floor with my head over the dirty toilet, dry heaving relentlessly, and he just walked out, got in the car, and went to his game. I was so angry and upset, it made me even sicker. —ANN F.

I think the biggest "sin of the husbands" is to not give the experience of morning sickness the credence it deserves. Don't ignore it. *Yes,* it *is* that bad. And yet many husbands have trouble understanding it. In fact, poor support by the partner was a complaint of 85 percent of women who called a morning sickness hotline.

It was a period of depression and struggle. I felt lazy 'cause I was unable to take care of my bills. My boyfriend felt tied down and it was hard, and that took a toll on our relationship. It was a big stress factor for both of us. —LYNETTE F.

Poor support by the partner was a complaint of 85 percent of women who called a morning-sickness hotline.

Above all, the partners of women with morning sickness should *educate* themselves. Look at it this way: if your wife had a chronic disease, you would hit the books, the Internet, the journals, and find the best doctors—to try to understand the illness and make sure she was in good hands—wouldn't you? Morning sickness should be no different. By finding out all you can about it, you will be more sympathetic to the realities.

He was very patient with my inability to eat foods that I used to enjoy. He would often come home from work with foods that I could eat and wouldn't complain about ordering in so frequently when I just couldn't prepare a meal.   —LAURA P.

Finding ways to help can be difficult of course, because every woman is different. Some like to be coddled and cuddled. Others prefer to be left alone. My poor husband Jon would ask almost every day if there was anything he could do, and the truth was, there wasn't. The last thing I wanted was someone hovering over me and asking to hold my hair back while I lost my lunch. But it made me feel *a lot* better that he cared to ask. In fact, Jon was the person who suggested I include a chapter on what partners should do, because he had felt so helpless most of the time.

When there were things he could do, like take me out for a steak, leave all spices out of his cooking for nine months, or let me lie down for two hours on a Saturday afternoon, I didn't hesitate to ask. And you shouldn't either. I'm not saying that you should demand to be spoiled and indulged for nine months; that's unrealistic, and it's likely to breed resentment in the most adoring of men. But, men, your mission, should you choose to accept it, is to be as considerate and patient as is humanly possible. You might have to give up your cologne for a little while, do more housework than usual, and forego the slobbery beer kisses you want to deliver after a night out with the boys—and *please*, NO CIGARS!

Men, your mission, should you choose to accept it, is to be as considerate as is humanly possible. Give up your cologne, do more housework than usual—and please, NO CIGARS!

My husband was on a diet and thus quite cranky. He decided to cook brussels sprouts, cauliflower, and broccoli all at the same time. I begged him to stop . . . he went on steaming those veggies. The house took on the aroma of those three horrors and I ran around and opened every window and dusted all the carpets with "I Love My Carpet" and vacuumed until the stench receded.

—LAURA P.

Maybe the moral of the story is: Keep the air clear . . . and the air will be clear between you. It may seem like forever, but it's a short-lived nod to the mother of your child, who would do the same for you. We like to think so, anyway.

12

The Vomit Chronicles

Get up, vomit. Shower, vomit. Brush teeth, vomit.
—CLAUDIA O'C.

Many women have told me they prefer not to dwell on other people's horror stories of morning sickness lest it bring on a tidal wave of nausea and make the whole experience even worse. For many, just talking about vomiting tends to bring on that sympathetic urge. If you're one of those women, skip this chapter. The whole point of this book is to make people feel better, not worse, but I did want to include these stories as a testament to survival. They are a glimpse of the incredibly difficult days we have all been through and yet have taken in stride and some of us can now laugh at. They are, for lack of a more delicate description, The Vomit Chronicles.

I didn't receive many responses to queries on this topic, perhaps because many women simply block it all out, or maybe because there are so many "worst days" that nothing stands out. I had that problem. Was it the time I was interviewing the dean of medicine at New York Hospital about heart disease when I started salivating, sweating, and praying, and had to rip off my microphone and bolt from the room? (The camera crews are *still* talking about it.) The time I vomited watermelon all over my office wall from about six feet away? Or maybe it was the Fourth of July, when we stood on the banks of the Hudson River waiting for the majestic tall ships to roll up and there I was, barfing in the bushes amidst hundreds and hundreds of people, and cannons being fired from the bows of the boats? To this day, when we walk past that site my daughter Noelle says, "Mommy, remember when you threw up here?"

Aaahh, the memories. Here are a few other unforgettable moments from fellow morning sickness sufferers.

I was driving in L.A. on the 405 in the morning rush hour to a meeting. I felt an incredible nausea sweeping over me and I realized I had to throw up. I had to pull over four lanes to the side of the road, where I proceeded to throw up with thousands of cars passing me through the L.A. smog. I never made it to the meeting, and had to return to the hotel and rest. —MIA K.

My husband was producing concerts in the park, and I had spent the day, hot and dusty, at the concert . . . there was a BBQ. I finally decided to go home I was so tired. Everyone insisted I take a taxi back to Brooklyn. During the ride, I discovered that being in the backseat of a cab made me instantly sick. So when we got to the Brooklyn Bridge, I threw up in the cab. Then I walked home and took the subway until the morning sickness passed.   —JENNY L.

I was pregnant with my daughter. I was at work and had been sick all day. Just as I was making a mad dash for the bathroom, I saw a man coming to the front door with a clipboard. I knew exactly who he was: the Salon State Inspector! After a five-minute stint throwing up, I came out and begged him to go away, but he refused. Men just don't understand.   —RAQUEL T.

We went out for dinner, where I actually felt like eating for a change and the food tasted good. So I ate, with gusto—veal parmigiana of all things, and Italian bread with butter. When we got home, I was so sick I didn't know if I should sit on or bend over the toilet bowl. I ended up sitting, but holding my head over the bathroom sink at the same time. Dinner was spouting uncontrollably into both bathroom fixtures. It was very glamorous. The whole morning-sickness/ pregnancy thing is so humbling. Once I had modesty. By the end, I couldn't care less if the New York Giants paraded through the delivery room as long as I got the whole thing over with.   —MARY JANE C.

I got dressed and got into the car with my husband and we drove to the train station. This was our usual routine. Not this particular day. My husband took a bath in aftershave cologne, or so it seemed. I rode to the train station with my head out the passenger window. We got to the station and the train had arrived early. My husband and I ran for it. We barely made it and I thought I was going to throw up or give birth. The woman to my right smelled of cheap, old lipstick, and the woman to the left of me reeked of old perfume. The conductor asked me for my train ticket as the odor of coffee hit my face. The next thing I remember was my husband standing over me, fanning me, calling my name. I had fainted. How embarrassing!   —ELIZABETH G.

I had a craving for poached salmon with green sauce. My husband, wanting to be accommodating, drove from our loft in Greenwich Village uptown to the Rosedale fish market during rush hour. When he returned with the fish, I was nauseated at the sight and smell of it . . . could not go near it."   —RUTH K.

I got sick in Home Depot . . . couldn't hold it."
     —JUNE N.

I just remember an image of myself walking through a food court in a mall and smelling all the aromas of the hot food and telling myself, "Oh, my God! Please get me out of here. This is making me sick! —DINA L.

I was running our newsroom's election coverage at the Democratic National Convention in Atlanta in 1988, and I was sick as a dog. Eighteen-hour days with an anchorman, reporters, crews, stories, press passes, pieces, problems. It was grueling work and the bath-room was miles away. Finally, toward the end of the day, our lead producer noticed I was eating Saltines and commented that she was eating them, too. We both looked quizzically at each other and said simul-taneously, "Are you . . . ?" We were. We felt great that both of us had kept it secret from each other while working under such difficult and pressure-filled cir-cumstances for nearly a week. We figured if we hadn't noticed each other, then surely the guys hadn't noticed us. We felt proud for women. Heck, you could be preg-nant and be in a pressure cooker, too." —SUSAN S.

I was at breakfast with the school-district superintend-ent and I thought I was going to throw up right there in front of thirty people. I made it back to school but ended up hugging the toilet bowl five minutes before I had to go teach for two hours, while the New York City School Board president was visiting our school."

—NICKY R.

I vomited in public in ShopRite after passing the fresh-fish counter. The store had such a combination of food smells, e.g.: rotisserie chickens, baking fish . . . I lost it. I felt as if the walls were caving in on me. I lost my peripheral vision, started sweating and salivating, and threw up within seconds. I was mortified!

—AMY C.

I once dashed between two parked cars on a quiet cross street with no one around . . . retch and run.

—EVA L.

Well, at the end of my twelfth week, I had my usual routine going until . . . I felt really really ill. I barely made it to the bathroom and boom! *Projectile vomiting right into the bowl. I felt better afterward. It was sort of like a swan song for my morning sickness.*

—HILARY T.

I took my son to the pool on a steamy day in June when I could not stay in our house another second because the carpets smelled, the laundry smelled, and the kitchen sink smelled, and the newspaper smelled . . . and I was so overcome by nausea at the pool that I squatted next to my son, who was digging in the soil by the bushes, and grabbed his shirt so he wouldn't wander to the water while I threw up in the bushes inconspicuously. Ugh.

—LU H.

. . . driving in Italy along hairpin turns in the mountains with a mixture of vomiting and diarrhea every half hour. I thought I needed a hospital but settled into a hotel to recover.

—MARY G.

It was my birthday and my husband selected a cozy, romantic, theater-row restaurant where we were to eat dinner before going to a show. The restaurant only offered a prix-fixe theater dinner at the hour we went and the choices were limited. Ordinarily, I would have been able to select at least one dish, but everything was so elaborately prepared and exotic that I nearly gagged just thinking about it. I wound up ordering salmon with no sauce, but between the appetizer and exotic salad, I felt slightly uncomfortable. By the time the meal was over, when we got to the theater and the show started, I felt much worse. At intermission, we decided to leave because I felt like I would really throw up. It wasn't such a fun evening.   —LAURA P.

One day on the way to work (7 A.M.), I was on the subway downtown and at about the Canal Street station I couldn't hold it anymore, so I got off the train, went outside, threw up in a garbage can, felt better, and got back on the train to go to work.   —KYOKO H.

After dinner at a restaurant, I threw up outside my house on the way home. Then it snowed. Then it thawed, and my husband teased me every day in spring as we could see the stain change and evolve and never quite go entirely away.   —SARAH D.

Is there a way to prevent these incidents? Probably not. As we've already established, we can't just remove ourselves from the world when we have morning sickness and we have to deal with our nausea in a very public way. But the one good thing I found about vomiting (the bright side of vomiting . . . now there's a concept) is that there *are* warning signs. Most of us know when we are going to lose it. We get sweaty, dizzy, clammy, and those salivary glands start working overtime. For me, the signs were a five-minute warning telling me: drop what you're doing, get up and leave the room, explain later.

Listen carefully to your body and it will tell you when to remove yourself from polite society. And if you don't make it, as embarrassing as it is, people (with the exception, maybe, of taxi drivers) will understand. Chances are that there's another woman witnessing your plight who's been in your shoes.

13

What to Pack
for the Journey

Though it may not seem imaginable from this vantage point, surviving morning sickness can be done. In some ways, just like labor and delivery, it is nothing more than a physical test requiring training, preparation, and endurance. In fact, it may help you to think of it that way, especially because every marathon has a finish line.

This is not to say that training and preparing for the marathon aren't challenging. Morning sickness demands a plan—a strategy—for outsmarting your body and letting you feel in better control. To do that, you will need some basic tools, a Morning-Sickness Survival Kit to be carried with you at all times. I am going to offer you a few ideas and suggestions, but you should personalize your own survival kit once you discover what your needs are.

To start with, you will need a bigger bag. That may not be possible since most women I know *already* hoist around luggage poorly disguised as a purse. But use this as an opportunity to get yourself a special morning-sickness tote or a nice backpack, something roomy enough to accommodate your needs. If you are feeling lousy, a little shopping excursion might cheer you up, anyway. You may never want to see this bag again once the need for it goes away, but I am sure it will hang stoically in your closet for years, a veteran of the morning-sickness wars.

Morning sickness demands a plan—a strategy—for outsmarting your body and letting you feel in better control.

The first thing you might want to start collecting is some of those air-sickness bags from airplanes. I know it sounds silly, but having a couple of them in your survival kit could save you some embarassment, and if nothing else, provide you with a security blanket. Given my history of motion sickness, I always check my seat pocket whenever I get on a plane just to make sure I have one. Somehow, it always makes me feel a little more relaxed to see it. So the next time you fly, just gather a couple, or ask the flight attendant for extras. You never know . . . and if you're not planning to fly during your pregnancy, maybe a friend who is could pick up several for you.

We have already discussed the need to have food with you at all times, and that is where you should begin. Never leave home without stowing something in your kit to snack on and drink. I recommend a bottle of water, a can of Coke or ginger ale, or both. Above all, you want to avoid getting dehydrated if you are vomiting, but you also might want to have something to sip that could stave off an episode of vomiting if you are on the brink. Something sugary and carbonated can often do the trick. If juice is your tonic, pack that along instead.

You'll also need a couple of different snacks to appeal to your fickle tastes. If you don't want to stuff your new purse like a grocery bag, I recommend buying plastic Ziploc (you can even get small, snack-sized ones) and filling them with a variety of comfort foods. Remember, think salty, sweet, crunchy, soft, to satisfy any craving. The following are portable, fairly nutritious, and could save you in a tight spot.

- PRETZELS
- WHOLE-WHEAT CRACKERS WITH OR WITHOUT PEANUT BUTTER. (I loved the pre-packaged peanut butter or cheese sandwich crackers that come six to a pack. They are not as healthy as

homemade because they are processed, but remember, check the guilt and go for convenience.)

- CARROTS AND CELERY STICKS. (Those baby carrots are easy to prepare.)
- APPLE SLICES
- AN ORANGE
- RICE CAKES
- GRAHAM CRACKERS
- NUTS: EITHER ROASTED ALMONDS OR PEANUTS
- YOUR FAVORITE CEREAL
- PACK ALONG A SPOON AND A SMALL YOGURT (if you're not going to be gone long and it won't get too warm).

There will of course be those times when you can't prevent vomiting no matter what's in your purse. Whether at the office or on the street, you will need some equipment to get you through it. Let's face it, vomiting leaves an awful taste in the mouth. Having water along will give you something to rinse your mouth with, but you might also want to carry a toothbrush and a travel toothpaste or mouthwash. If brushing your teeth makes you nauseous, try mints, hard candies, or gum. Anything you can find to clear the taste out of your mouth and make you feel fresher will be helpful. And speaking of feeling fresher, I also recommend that you carry along some wet wipes such as baby wipes or Handi Wipes. They often come in little individually wrapped packets and smell clean and refreshing; cleaning

Above all, you want to avoid getting dehydrated if you are vomiting, but you also might want to have something to sip that could stave off an episode of vomiting if you are on the brink.

your hands and face and rubbing one over the back of your neck will help restore you to humanity. If you can't stand any scents or fragrances at all, many wet wipes come unscented as well. And don't forget to pack some of those travel packs of tissue. They are handy for a million reasons, not the least of which will be wiping the occasional tear away when you feel you can't take it anymore!

Finally, let me throw in one last self-serving suggestion to help you get through the days. Throw this little book in your bag so that you can read the next chapter, "A Little Advice from the Experts," over and over again during moments of weakness. My hope is that the quotes and thoughts from fellow sufferers will be a big help, providing you with a dose of stamina, insight, humor, and patience with yourself: the most important things to have in your survival kit.

14

A Little Advice from the Experts

Some family members would tell me, "Just get up and take a walk, or go outside," and I would want to strangle them.
                                                    —LORI S.

When I was in the thick of it, walking through the days in slow motion, wondering why in the world I wanted to have another child, people pushing advice drove me crazy. Yeah, yeah, yeah, I would say sarcastically, I have heard it all before. Suuuurrre, crackers don't work, but rice cakes and matzoh are going to save me. I guess I felt that no one could know how I felt, and therefore, no one could help me in any way. Well, that was a little short-sighted obviously, but I would be the first to admit that I was feeling a little sorry for myself at the time.

Without any time-tested remedies on the market, managing your morning sickness is all about trial and error, as we saw in the chapter dealing with food. It's also about being your own pep rally and cheerleading squad. Just as the symptoms can get you down, you have to find ways to rally and fight back. So with that in mind, I want to include some of the pearls of wisdom your fellow sufferers have offered. I have tried to include short and pithy thoughts so you can close your eyes and repeat them over and over like a mantra on particularly bad days if you need to. Some address physical problems, others offer mental and emotional support. All are intended to help you find something new to at least try without saying what I did: yeah, yeah, yeah . . .

Don't sniff any leftovers.   —PAT L.

Don't be afraid to eat. . . . It may really be hunger pangs that feel the same as morning sickness.
                                        —KAREN T.

Try sucking on ice chips.   —ELLA D.

It will invariably end, and you won't remember much about it later. . . .   —SUSAN R.

Food does not make it go away . . . so don't over indulge.   —HILARY R.T.

Keep in mind that the nausea means the pregnancy is progressing normally.   —LAURA P.

Keep busy so you don't have time to think about it and feel sorry for yourself. —JULIE S.

It can be really bad and if you don't have morning sickness, don't brag about it. We are happy for you but it just makes those of us who are suffering so badly feel worse. —SUSAN S.

Eat turkey tetrazzini and find one woman who has been through it to share your feelings with. That is the big lifesaver. —PAXTON B.

I only hope that every woman who is pregnant and suffering from morning sickness finds a kindred spirit to comfort her during this extremely trying time. —CHRISTINE H.

Literally: "One day at a time." —LORI S.

Keep eating tiny bits of protein constantly. —ANONYMOUS

Get sleep! Beg, borrow, steal to have others care for already-existing kids so you can nap or sleep in. —LOUISA W.

Ginger! I ate ginger snaps compulsively on car trips. —CARYN R.

Don't try to do too much. —MEG G.

Follow your cravings.   —JODIE G.

Keep the big picture in mind. Remember, the whole point is that you'll have a child forever after.

—JULIE

Eat often, eat small portions of small food.

—ANNE P.

Try sipping Coke or ginger ale all throughout the day.

—MICHELLE

Try everything with the help of a good doctor.

—ANATILDE G.

Don't try to get through it alone.   —JENNY L.

. . . It is not a reflection on you, your strength as a person, nor your psychological state or abilities as a mother.   —MARY G.

I am sure that the way you handle stress has a lot to do with how you feel during pregnancy . . . get serious about the way you handle stresses in your life and put a plan into place.   —ANN C.

Toss guilt out the window, and eat gooey french onion soup for three days if it's what your body is begging for. No craving is permanent, and fulfilling cravings is not detrimental to you or your baby. . . .   —LU H.

The sense that my body and baby were healthy in spite of my feeling horrible was, in fact, a comfort to me.
                                                —EVA L.

Mints! I always sucked on mints!   —MICHELLE B.

Space your children apart . . . it's hard to nap with a baby.   —RAQUEL T.

Take care of yourself! Indulge in as much rest, relaxation, sleep, bathing, meditation, and otherwise stress-relieving activities as possible. Don't become overtired.
                                                —CHRIS S.

Keep remembering that suffering can build character.
                                                —AMY C.

Listen to your body and what feels right for you. I believe that will be the right thing for your baby, too.
                                                —NICKY R.

Just hang in there! It gets better and in the end, it's all worth it.   —JUNE N.

Try to accept it as part of the miracle.   —IRENE K.

Take the huge pink prenatal vitamin with food at the end of the day. Maybe you, too, can sleep through the nausea.   —SUE P.

Try to keep as much fluid in your body as possible so dehydration doesn't set in.   —LYNNETTE F.

It's not terminal!   —RUTH S. K.

Try to rethink any negative attitudes . . . the nausea is proof positive that you're creating a life.
          —HEATHER S.

Despite what you might think, you are not a freak. *Honey, everything you are experiencing is real and you don't have to make little of how miserable it is.*
          —MARY JANE C.

Humor . . . endure . . . It prepares you for the trials of parenthood.   —GEORGETTE D.

Don't dwell on not feeling good.   —DONNA B.

Keep your eye on the prize: the baby.   —LAURA P.

15

The Future: New Thinking About an Old Problem

By now, you know that there's an unfortunate cloud of ennui hovering over the problem of morning sickness. The ailment has been around forever, but as we've learned, there's little groundbreaking research on the topic. You'd think scientists would love to tackle an unsolved medical mystery, especially one that has such a profound impact on the daily lives of women who go through it. But few people are interested in taking it on, except of course the women who have it, and as a result, too many conversations about morning sickness begin and end in five minutes. Usually, crackers are mentioned.

I wish I could report that in the course of writing this

book, I tapped into what the great minds of obstetric medicine are learning about the problem in all the hundreds of trials and studies being done. I wish I could tell you that we will unlock the mystery of morning sickness in the next few years and solve it. But I'm not confident of that.

Before you throw up (no pun intended) your hands in despair, there is some hope. There is a small community of people—doctors and researchers—feverishly focused on the subject, and as a result, there *is* progress to report; some new thinking about this old problem that may benefit your daughters and your granddaughters.

First of all, there is an evolving understanding in the medical community of what morning sickness is. Some researchers are beginning to look at it as a *syndrome*. In other words, it's not just about nausea and vomiting, but involves a whole list of discrete mechanisms, and women will suffer depending on their varying degrees of susceptibility to these mechanisms. The belief now is that morning

The belief now is that morning sickness is the product of a whole domino effect of predispositions: genetics, age, susceptibility to motion sickness, vestibular dysfunction of the inner ear, a tendency to sensitivity to smells or tastes, and a proclivity for having migraines.

sickness is the product of a whole domino effect of predis-positions: genetics, age, susceptibility to motion sickness, vestibular dysfunction of the inner ear, a tendency to be sensitive to smells or tastes (doctors call it being a hyper-taster!), and a proclivity for having migraines, all wrapped up in one big package. There are estimates that 10 to 20 percent of the population are walking around with one or more of these tendencies, and if you then add a healthy dose of HCG, estrogen, and progesterone—voila! Morning sickness in all its varying degrees.

It turns out that many women with a tendency toward motion sickness also have morning sickness.

I find this thinking fascinating because I have always suffered terrible *motion* sickness. I can't read in cars, don't get on boats without Dramamine, and even if you offered me large sums of money, would not get in that twirling teacup ride at the amusement park. Memories of whale-watching expeditions and chopper rides I had to take for work give me vertigo. So I have always wondered if my tendency toward motion sickness was at all related to my bad bouts of morning sickness. Is it a weak stomach or an inner-ear problem? Or a combination of both? It turns out that many women with a tendency toward motion sickness also have morning sickness. We don't know why, but that the link exists even anecdotally raises interesting questions worth exploring. If we could understand the mechanism linking morning and motion sicknesses, or why some people have more acute senses of smell and taste than other people, we might get to the heart of what causes morning sickness and, in turn, know how to treat it better. Not suppress it, just treat it better. More research needs to be done in these areas.

Much of the research on morning sickness is being done in Canada. That's the home of the drug company Duchesnay, which manufactures Diclectin, and the headquarters of the organization Motherisk, which is affiliated with the Hospital for Sick Children in Toronto. Duchesnay sets aside 20 percent of its annual revenues to fund a wide range of projects involving pregnant women and morning sickness, and as I mentioned, is working hard with the FDA to bring Diclectin to the United States.

Motherisk is also involved in a lot of research aimed at trying to quantify morning sickness so that it can be better understood. To that end, doctors working at Motherisk have developed a new tool for measuring the severity of nausea and vomiting. Because we all have to maintain our sense of humor, the tool is called the P.U.Q.E and is pronounced "puke." It stands for Pregnancy Unique Quantification of Emesis—"Unique" because it does not measure nausea in people undergoing chemotherapy, for example. And emesis, by now you know, means vomiting. The new tool measures three symptoms in women with morning sickness: number of times of vomiting per day, number of hours of nausea, and number of bouts of retching. By gathering this sort of data, scientists will be able to amass a body of knowledge that has never existed before, detailing varying degrees of morning sickness and potentially guiding them toward better treatment and prevention.

Motherisk is also focused on pulling back the curtain that has hidden the emotional and psychological burdens of morning sickness for so long. Although the organization generally deals with the worst cases of *Hyperemesis Gravidarum,* Motherisk's morning-sickness hotline fields as many as two hundred phone calls a day from women needing counseling and support. Proof positive that morning sickness is not just about nausea! That information is also contributing to a growing body of scientific knowledge that can only help us all in our understanding of morning sickness.

And one final piece of good news: understanding and treating nausea and vomiting in pregnancy is about to become part of the curriculum for the thousands of people training to be obstetricians and gynecologists. Just this

Motherisk's morning sickness hotline fields as many as 200 phone calls a day from women needing counseling and support. Proof positive that morning sickness is not just about nausea!

year, the Association of Professors of Gynecology and Obstetrics, along with the American College of Obstetricians and Gynecologists, drafted what they call a "teaching monograph" of morning sickness, a lesson plan designed to help medical-school faculty who want to teach the subject. Morning Sickness will now join a list of fourteen other high-profile, high-interest, health-care issues facing women today that are being discussed in the classroom. Cardiovascular disease, contraception, osteoporosis, and premenstrual syndrome are just a few of the other concerns on the list. The "teaching monograph" will also be distributed to the thirty-eight thousand practicing members of the American College of Obstetrics and Gynecology.

It's about time, don't you think? Now a whole new generation of doctors will have a greater understanding of the totality of morning sickness, advising you not only on how to keep food down, but how to keep your job, keep your marriage, your sanity, and care for your other children.

It may well be that we will never have a cure or the perfect treatment for morning sickness. We may never pin down its exact cause. But a broader understanding of what it is, and the wide variety of ways it affects us, will go a long way toward making easier the lives of women who suffer through it. Thankfully, the research is now taking quality of life into consideration and is breaking new ground in our comprehension of morning sickness. The progress isn't seismic, but it's there, and we'll all be better off for it.

Epilogue:
Some Final Thoughts

I felt great about myself. Here was proof that we were creating a baby together. As vile as the physical sensations were, I wouldn't trade experiencing any of it.

—HEATHER S.

I am writing this book with the safety and clarity that a little distance provides. My son is now six months old. It has been a year since I sat drained, despondent, and miserable on the bathroom floor in front of the toilet bowl wondering when my anguish would end and if I would survive it.

I don't really remember the day-to-day feeling: coffee tastes just as delicious to me as it always did, and salad is once again my favorite lunch. And yet the experience of morning sickness was so traumatic that I felt compelled to write about it. I may not be there anymore, but I will never forget those days.

The good news is that there is a happy ending here. I can laugh about things now that you may have a lot of trouble finding funny. I can file the whole experience away as one of life's curiosities and struggles, whereas you may not believe you can get through another day. And most important, I can watch my baby boy crack a mile-wide, toothless grin, and beam with pride as my little girl learns to write her name. I mean, no wonder I felt so horrible: look at how incredible they are! Was I expecting the creation of these complex, intricate, beautiful little individuals to be easy? I know without a shadow of a doubt that I would go through the whole nightmare again to have them in my life.

I don't mean to sound glib about how bad the whole thing is by saying, "Oh, what's four months of nausea and vomiting when you get a baby out of the deal?" I am particularly sensitive to the plight of those women with the extreme form of morning sickness, *Hyperemesis Gravidarum*. For them, even the payoff becomes questionable, and that's very real. But for me, and I am hoping for you, too, what it boils down to is a tough lesson learned: there are a few things in life worth such struggle, and children top the list.

Your bout with morning sickness will always provide you with powerful memories and a profound sense of relief and accomplishment. But it will also give you something much bigger that you may not have considered: your first reminder that motherhood is full of challenges that yield great joy. It's a test that involves strength and stamina, grace and humor, patience and love. Oh, and a good doctor. The very tools you will need to raise your children, you may have already mastered, just by surviving morning sickness.

Bibliography

Erick, Miriam. *No More Morning Sickness: A Survival Guide for Pregnant Women*. New York: Penguin Books, 1993.

Koren, Gideon, and Bishai Raafat, et al. *Nausea and Vomiting of Pregnancy: State of the Art 2000*. Toronto, Canada: Motherisk, The Hospital for Sick Children, 2000.

Park, Robert L. *Voodoo Science: The Road from Foolishness to Fraud*. New York: Oxford Univ. Press, 2000.

Profet, Margie. *Pregnancy Sickness: Using Your Body's Natural Defenses to Protect Your Baby-To-Be*. Boston: Addison Wesley, 1995.

Soranus. *Soranus Gynecology*. Translated by Owsei Temkin. Baltimore and London: Johns Hopkins Univ. Press, 1956.

INDEX